ICD-10-CM External Cause Coding Made Easy

2021

Terry Tropin, MSHAI, RHIA, CCS-P

AHIMA-Approved ICD-10-CM/PCS Trainer

REVIEWERS

Aylin Edelman, MD, RHIT, CCS
Health Information Specialist

Suzanne Lasky, CPC

Lauren Pitts, MHA, RHIA, CCS, CCS-P
3M Health Information Systems
Clinical Development Analyst

Tasha E. Green, MS, RHIA, CHTS-TR, FAHIMA
AHIMA Certified ICD-10 Trainer
Program Director and Associate Professor
Health Information Management Department
Prince George's Community College
Largo, Maryland

Miroslava Rudneva, RHIT, CCS

To Zee – Who always provides unfailing support

Table of Contents

Introduction 5
PART 1 - ICD-10-CM CHANGES FOR 2021 7
PART 2 - EXTERNAL CAUSE DEFINITIONS 9
Transportation Accidents 9
Definitions - External Causes for Transport Accidents V00-V99 9
Definitions - Patient Status in Transport Accidents... 10
Transportation Accidents: Definitions of Vehicles 10
Nontransportation Accident Definitions.. 13
Terms Related to Treatment/After-Effects of Treatment... 14
Terms Related to Devices 15
PART 3 - EXTERNAL CAUSE OF INJURIES - CODING GUIDELINES 17
General Coding Guidelines... 17
Coding Guidelines for Injury and External Cause Codes 18
Coding Guidelines for Other Specific Circumstances... 19
PART 4 - FINDING EXTERNAL CAUSE CODES 21
Categories of External Causes 22
Finding External Cause Codes – Which, What, Who, When, Where 23
Category Of Intent/Cause - Accidents 24
Category Of Intent/Cause - Nonaccidents 36
      Assault 36
      Legal Intervention 40
      Terrorism 42
      Undetermined... 44
Category of Intent/Cause - Military 45
Category – Medical Treatment/Complication 49
      Misadventure 49
      Injuries Related to Adverse reaction to medical devices 50
      Injuries Related to Abnormal reaction to Medical Treatment 50

PART 5 - INDEX OF EXTERNAL CAUSE OF INJURIES ... 53

Activity Codes ... 54
Place of Occurrence ... 58
Status of External Cause ... 63
Category – Intent/Cause - Accidents - Transport ... 64
- Air and Space Vehicles ... 64
- Land – Nontraffic ... 66
- Land – Traffic ... 91
- Land – Unspecified as Traffic or Nontraffic ... 116
- Watercraft ... 119

Category – Intent/Cause - Accidents - Other ... 126
Category – Intent/Cause - Nonaccidents ... 145
- Assault ... 145
- Legal Intervention ... 148
- Self-harm ... 151
- Terrorism ... 153
- Undetermined ... 155

Category – Intent/Cause - Military ... 157
- Military Operations ... 157
- War Operations ... 160

Category - Intent/Cause - Medical Treatment/Complications ... 164
- Adverse Incidents Associated with Devices ... 164
- Complications of medical/surgical treatment ... 166
- Misadventures ... 167

Sequelae ... 169
Supplemental Factors ... 169

Introduction

Many coders find the Official Coding Guidelines for ICD-10-CM external cause codes dense, confusing, and repetitive. In addition, terms such as animate mechanical forces, controlled fire, and conflagration are not defined. Other definitions are buried within the guidelines and difficult to locate. Finally, the index to external causes is long, very confusing and hard to follow.

Conditions related to transport accidents may be found in other sections. For example, injury due to an airbag (W22.1-) and injury to due rupture of bicycle tire (W37.0) are in the section Exposure to Inanimate Mechanical Forces, not transport accidents.

Entries can be confusing. For example, the Alphabetic Index references code V19.88- to report entanglement of clothing in pedal wheel. However, in the Tabular List, this code is defined as another specified cyclist accident.

This publication addresses the problems described above. Also, the index is reorganized and related codes are grouped together. This book is based on the codes and guidelines from the 2021 Official Coding Guidelines, released October 2020.

It is designed for use as a supplement to coding textbooks for students and as a quick reference for coders working in the field. It clarifies the external cause guidelines using charts to provide step by step directions on how to interpret the guidelines, including codes, definitions and sequencing. Coders should confirm the code selected using the Tabular List in the ICD-10-CM code book.

The book consists of five parts:
- ICD-10-CM Changes for 2021
- Definitions of terms
- Guidelines for selecting codes for external causes of morbidity
- Finding external cause codes – What, Why, Who, How, Which, When and Where
- Simplified external cause of injuries index

Part 1
ICD-10-CM Changes for 2021

Following is a summary of the changes in ICD-10-PCS effective October 1, 2020. For complete list of changes to ICD-10-CM, see
https://www.cms.gov/Medicare/Coding/ICD10/2021-ICD-10-CM.html

Added hoverboard, Segway, standing electric scooter, standing micro-mobility pedestrian conveyance to these sections:
- Pedestrian conveyance accident V00
- Collision with pedal cycle V01
- Two- or three-wheeled motor vehicle V02
- Collision with car, pick-up truck or van V03
- Heavy transport vehicle or bus V04
- Railway train or railway vehicle V05
- Other nonmotor vehicle V06

Other new codes are:
- Y77.11 contact lens associated with adverse incidents
- Y77.19 Other therapeutic (nonsurgical) and rehabilitative ophthalmic devices associated with adverse incidents

Part 2
External Cause Definitions

Transportation Accidents

Following are definitions of terms used in the External Causes of Morbidity chapter.

Definitions - External Causes for Transport Accidents V00-V99 *

Terms	Definitions
Transport accident	Involves vehicle designed primarily for, or used at the time of the accident primarily for, moving persons or goods from one place to another. Vehicle is moving, running or in use at the time of the accident.
Patient in transport accident	Patient may be: pedestrian injured by vehicle; using a pedestrian conveyance; or in or on a vehicle (driver, passenger or hanger-on).
Boarding or alighting	Boarding: getting into/on vehicle Alighting: getting out of/off vehicle
Collision	Vehicle collides with (hits) another vehicle, person, or fixed or stationary object.
Noncollision	Vehicle does **NOT** collide (hit) with another vehicle, person, fixed or stationary object. Example: • Car overturns due to ice on road. • Vehicle has mechanical problem leading to injury. • Patient hit by vehicle while stopped on side of road to change tire.
Nontraffic accident	Accident did not occur on public highway. Occurred on private road, driveway, or off-road.
Traffic accident	Accident on public highway. Vehicle started or ended partly or completely on public highway.
Public highway**	Entire span of road from one boundary line to the other. Includes shoulders or dividers in highway. Area open to public.
Roadway	Part of public highway used for traffic (not including shoulders or dividers).

*Assume transport injury was accidental unless documented otherwise.
**Assume the accident was on a public highway if not otherwise specified except for accident involving all-terrain vehicle.

Codes list first the patient's means of transportation and then other vehicle involved. Example: Patient in car has accident with dump truck. External Cause Index: Accident, transport, car, collision, with pickup truck (V43.93).

Patient in vehicle may be described as: driver, passenger, hanger-on or occupant. Other patients may be pedestrians or using a pedestrian conveyance. These are defined as follows:

Definitions - Patient Status in Transport Accidents

Patient status	Definitions
Driver	Patient was operating or intending to operate vehicle.
Passenger	Patient was inside vehicle but was not driving.
Hanger-on	Patient was not inside vehicle. May be hanging onto bumper, fender, roof, running board or step of vehicle.
Occupant	Patient not identified as driver, hanger-on or passenger OR No specific code for driver, hanger-on or passenger is listed.*
Pedestrian	Patient not in vehicle or hanging on to any part of a vehicle. Patient may be on side of road changing tire, working on car or walking.
Using pedestrian conveyance	Patient pushing a baby carriage, on ice skates, roller skates, skateboard, hoverboard, Segway, nonmotorized or motorized wheelchair or scooter.

*Example: Bus passenger alighting bus collides with pedestrian. Use code V70.4 (person boarding or alighting a bus was injured in collision with pedestrian). No codes indicate whether patient alighting bus was passenger or driver of bus.

Transportation Accidents: Definitions of Vehicles

Type of Vehicle	Description	Examples
Agricultural vehicle V84	Carries goods Motorized Used in farming and agriculture to work the land, tend and harvest crops and transport materials.	Harvester Other farm machinery Tractor Trailers
Air and space vehicles V95-V97	Carries passengers or goods Nonmotorized or motorized	Airplanes Helicopters Gliders Hot-air balloon
All-terrain vehicle V86	Motorized Used to negotiate over rough or soft terrain, snow or sand.	All-terrain vehicles Dirt bikes Dune buggy Does **NOT** include sport utility vehicle (SUV). See van/pick-up truck
Animal being ridden V80	Person using animal as transportation	Horse rider, mule rider
Animal-drawn vehicle V80	Carries passengers or goods Nonmotorized	Horse-drawn carriage Mule cart
Bus V70-V79	Carries more than 10 passengers. Motorized Requires special driver's license.	City bus Motor coach Land coach School bus
Car V40-V49	Carries up to 7 people. Motorized. Four wheeled vehicle. Includes car being towed by trailer.	Automobile Does **NOT** include sport utility vehicle (SUV). See van/pick-up truck

Transportation Accidents: Definitions of Vehicles (continued)

Type of Vehicle	Description	Examples
Construction vehicle V85	Carries goods. Motorized. Used at construction and demolition sites.	Backhoes, Bulldozers, Diggers, Dump trucks, Earth-levelers, Front-end loaders, Mechanical shovels, Pavers. Does **NOT** include these vehicles when stationary use or in maintenance.
Heavy transport vehicle V60-V69	Carries goods. Motorized. Meets local weight criteria for classification as heavy goods vehicle. Requires a special driver's license.	Armored truck, Eighteen-wheeler, Panel truck. Does **NOT** include bus or pick-up truck
Industrial vehicle V83	Carries passengers or goods. Motorized. Used primarily within an industrial or commercial business (in a building).	Battery-powered trucks, Coal-cars in mine, Forklifts, Logging cars, Self-propelled industrial truck, Trucks used in mines or quarries
Military vehicle V86	Motorized. Operates on public roadway. Owned by military. Operator is member of military.	Tank. Any vehicle owned by military
Mobility scooter V00.83-	Motorized. 3 or 4 wheels.	Motorized mobility scooter
Motorcycle V20-V29	Motorized. Two wheels. One or two riding saddles. May have third wheel attached for sidecar.	Motorcycle, Motorized bicycle, Motor scooter, Two-wheeled vehicle with attached sidecar
Other and unspecified V98-V99	Vehicles that do not fit into other categories listed.	Cable car, Ski lift, Unspecified, Yacht
Pedal cycle V10-V19	Nonmotorized.	Bicycle, Tricycle, Rickshaw, Sidecar or trailer attached to pedal cycle
Pedestrian V00-V09	May be on foot or using pedestrian conveyance (such as roller skates).	
Pick-up truck V50-V59	Carriers passengers or property. Motorized. Four-six wheels. For property or cargo weighing less than the local limit for classification as heavy goods vehicle. Does not require special driver's license.	Minibus, Minivan, Sport utility vehicle (SUV), Truck, Van
Railway train or railway vehicle V81	Carries passengers or freight. Motorized – runs on railway track. May or may not have cars attached to it.	Elevated train, Subway, Train. Does **NOT** include streetcar. See V82
Rolling stock V81	Any vehicle (including self-propelled or pulled vehicle) used on a track.	Caboose, train car. Does **NOT** include streetcar. See V82.

Transportation Accidents: Definitions of Vehicles (continued)

Type of vehicle	Description	Examples
Standing micro-mobility pedestrian conveyance V0.84-	Motorized Travel at low speed Rider is upright (not sitting down)	Segway Standing electric scooter Hoverboard
Streetcar V82	Carries passengers. Motorized-runs on track. Runs within a municipality. Usually subject to normal traffic signals. Operates principally on roadway.	Streetcar — Trailer being towed by streetcar Tram — Does **NOT** include nonpowered streetcar or train Trolley
Three-wheeled vehicle V30-V39	Motorized. Used primarily on-road.	Motorized tricycle Motorized rickshaw Does NOT include all-terrain vehicle
Van V50-V59	Carriers passengers or property. Motorized. Four-six wheels. For property or cargo weighing less than the local limit for classification as heavy goods vehicle. Does not require special driver's license.	Truck Minibus Minivan Sport utility vehicle (SUV) Van
Watercraft V90-V94	Carries passengers or goods. Motorized or nonmotorized. Used on water.	Canoes Motorboats Sailboats Ships

Nontransportation Accident Definitions

Term	Definition	Examples
Terms Related to Fire/Flames X00-X08		
Conflagration	Fire that destroys large areas of land or property. Type of uncontrolled fire.	Forest fire Wildfire
Controlled fire	Fire or flame started for benign purpose (such as cooking or providing heat or light).	Campfire, bonfire, deliberately set trash fire, fireplace, stove
Uncontrolled fire	Fire started accidentally or in order to do harm.	Fire in a building or forest, furniture caught on fire by cigarette.
Ignition	Set on fire. Type of uncontrolled fire.	Nightgown set on fire by dropped cigarette
Terms Related to Military/Terrorism/Law Enforcement		
Legal intervention Y35	Injury due to contact with any law enforcement officer, on-duty or off-duty.	May be injury to law enforcement official, suspect or by-stander Injury due to firearm, Taser or baton
Military operations Y37	Injury to military and civilian personnel occurring during: • Peacetime on military property and/or • Routine military exercises and operations	Injury during basic training Slipping/falling in barracks in the U.S.
War operations Y36	Injury to military and civilian personnel during: • War • Civil insurrection and • Peacekeeping missions	Injury during war activities Slipping/falling while on patrol in hostile area
Perpetrator Y07	Person who injured patient.	Identified by relationship to patient (mother, brother, cousin, day care provider, etc.)
Terrorism Y38	Injury resulting from unlawful use of force or violence against persons or property to intimate or coerce a Government, the civilian population, or any segment thereof, in furtherance of political or social objectives.	9/11 Must be identified as terrorism by the FBI If not, use code for assault
Public safety official Y38	Includes law enforcement officer, firefighter, chaplain, or member of rescue squad or ambulance crew.	Used in codes for Terrorism
Terms Related to Weather or Natural Occurrences X30-X39		
Forces of nature	Weather-related and geological events	Snowstorm, flood, draught
Cataclysm	Large, destructive event involving forces of nature	Earthquake, volcano, tsunami, hurricane

(continued on next page)

Nontransportation Accident Definitions (continued)

Term	Definition	Examples
Other Terms		
Animate mechanical forces	Injury due to **living** being (person or animal).	Animal bite or human stampede
Inanimate mechanical forces	Injury due to **nonliving** object or machine.	Patient crushed between machines. Foot run over by power lawnmower
Foreign body	Something from the environment that is inside body – swallowed, in skin, inhaled, or inserted in orifice (body opening).	Gravel in a wound, penny inserted into nostril, bullet in abdomen, fish bone caught in throat, splinter in finger
Nosocomial	Condition acquired during hospitalization. May or may not be due to treatment.	Infection caught during hospital stay
Submersion (submerged)	Patient's head goes underwater, with or without subsequent drowning.	May be accidental, self-harm or due to assault
Intent	Reason the patient was injured	Accident, self-harm (suicide attempt), homicide, legal intervention, etc.
Undetermined intent	Physician documents that the intent (accidental, assault, or self-harm) cannot be determined.	Patient drove into wall. Physician documents that he cannot determine whether injury was accidental or suicide attempt

Terms Related to Treatment/After-Effects of Treatment*

Term	Definition	Examples
Complication	Surgical and medical procedure or device caused abnormal reaction. May be documented immediately after procedure or later. If due to physician error, see Misadventures	Hemorrhage following procedure. Sepsis following procedure
Device	Device - An instrument, apparatus, implement, machine, contrivance, implant, in vitro reagent, or other similar article. Its primary purpose is not achieved by a chemical action within or on the body or being metabolized within the body. See below for definitions of types of devices.	
Adverse incident due to device	Problem with device during use, after implantation, or during ongoing use	Pacemaker malfunction. Breakdown of device.
Abnormal reaction to treatment	Reaction may be to surgical or medical treatment. May be abnormal reaction or later complication. No misadventure at time of treatment	Pacemaker working normally; patient develops inflammation around it.
Misadventure	Injury or adverse effect resulting from medical treatment (due to physician error).	Accidental puncturing of organ during procedure. Sponge left in surgical wound.
Sequela (of)	Condition that is result of previous (treated) disease or (healed) injury. Treatment has been completed. Also referred to as late effects. Use code for original injury with 7th character S.	Scar. Abnormal gait after fracture treatment has been completed.

*Sometimes multiple codes are needed to completely describe the circumstances. See Excludes2 notes in categories Y62-Y84. For examples, see page 49.

Terms Related to Devices

Types of devices (used for complications/adverse incident/abnormal reaction)		
Term	**Definition**	**Examples**
Accessory device	Supports another device	Rechargeable battery for an automated external defibrillator
Diagnostic device	Determines patient's condition	Magnet resonance Imaging (MRI)
Miscellaneous device	Device that does not fall into any of the other categories listed	
Monitoring device	Tracks body functions	Pulse oximeters
Personal device	Device that may be used by patient outside of outpatient facility	Ice bag, body waste receptacle
Prosthetic device	Artificial body part that replaces missing body part	Hip replacement
Rehabilitative device	Helps improve functioning	Back brace
Surgical device and materials	Device or materials used during procedure	Endoscope, sutures
Therapeutic device	Treats patient's condition	Pacemaker

Part 3
External Cause of Injuries - Coding Guidelines

The primary code is the intent/cause of injury code. Locate the appropriate intent/cause code first. Other codes (activity, status of external causes, and place of occurrence) are also listed when appropriate.

General Coding Guidelines

Circumstances	Guidelines
Use of codes	Not required nationally. May be required by state or a specific payer. Never listed first on claim form.
Use with other codes	May be listed with any code A00.0-T88.9, Z00-Z99. Most often listed with injury codes.
Characters	Most codes have 7th characters. Many codes will require multiple X placeholders.
Multiple external cause codes	List as many as needed to fully describe circumstances. List most serious injury first. Claim form may limit number of codes that can be reported. List external cause codes in this order: • Child and adult abuse (X92-Y09) • Terrorism (Y38) • Cataclysmic events (earthquake, tsunami, hurricane, etc.) (X34-X38) • Transport accidents (V00-V99) • Activity (Y93) • External cause status (Y99)
Combination external cause codes	Codes that report sequential events that result in an injury (such as a fall through glass with resulting striking against an object). Injury does **NOT** need to be specifically linked to one event or the other (the fall or the striking against). Injury may be due to both events. Use the appropriate combination code regardless of which injury is more severe or occurred first.
Two or more events cause separate injuries	List external cause code for each event.
Transport injuries	Intent is assumed to be accidental. If injury documented as due to assault, see Assault, with subterms such as Struck by, Crash or Pushing. If injury documented as due to self-harm, see Suicide, with subterms such as Collision or Jumped.
Undetermined intent	Intent/cause of injury not documented. Physician must specifically document intent as undetermined.
Unknown intent	Code as accidental. All transport accidents are assumed to be accidental unless otherwise indicated.
Sequelae	Late effect resulting from previous injury. Use 7th character S on codes for original injury and external cause code. List these codes for subsequent visits for treatment of late effect of initial injury. Do **NOT** use S character on current condition. Do **NOT** list sequela codes for follow-up visits if no late effect is documented. Do **NOT** list external cause for sequelae with external cause for related current injury.

Coding Guidelines for Injury and External Cause Codes

Circumstances	Codes	When Code is Used	Comments
Use ALPHABETIC Index			
Injury or condition	A00-T88, Z00-Z99	List before external cause codes	
Use EXTERNAL CAUSE Index			
External cause codes listed throughout treatment – Intent/Cause of Injury			
Accidental	V00-X58	List before other external cause codes If more than one cause, list code for each. List external cause for most serious injury first.	Do **NOT** use for poisonings, adverse effects, underdosing or toxic effects.
Intentional self-harm	X71-X83		
Assault	X92-Y09		
Legal intervention	Y35		
Operations of war	Y36		
Military operations	Y37		
Terrorism	Y38	FBI must confirm event as act of terrorism.	Do **NOT** use if terrorism not confirmed by FBI. List code for assault instead.
Misadventures/ Complications	Y62-Y84	Medical device malfunctions or breaks down. Abnormal reaction to surgical or medical procedure.	
Undetermined	Y21-Y33	Physician documented that intent cannot be determined.	
External Cause Codes listed only for initial encounter			
Activity	Y93	List only one activity code. List with cause and intent codes.	Do **NOT** use for poisonings, adverse effects, underdosing, toxic effects, misadventures, subsequent visits or sequelae. Do **NOT** list Y93.9 if activity is not documented.
Status of patient	Y99	List only one status code. List whenever other external cause code used.	Do **NOT** use for poisonings, adverse effects, underdosing, toxic effects, misadventures, subsequent visits or sequelae. Do **NOT** use if no other external cause code is being listed. Do **NOT** list Y99.9 if status not documented.
Place of occurrence	Y92	List only one place of occurrence code. List after other external cause codes.	Do **NOT** use for poisonings, adverse effects, underdosing, toxic effects, misadventures, subsequent visits or sequelae. Do **NOT** list Y92.9 if no place of occurrence documented.

External cause codes are **NEVER** listed as principal diagnosis

For initial visit, list external cause codes in this order: Intent and cause; activity, status of patient, and place of occurrence (if information is available).

Coding Guidelines for Other Specific Circumstances

Circumstances	Coding Guidelines
Child or Adult Abuse*	
Confirmed	Provider must document abuse as confirmed. List first code T74-. Then list any mental health or injury codes. Then list external cause code for assault (X92-Y09). Then list code for perpetrator (person who injured patient) of the abuse if known (Y07).
Suspected	List first code T76-. Then list any mental health or injury codes. Then list Z04.7- (observation for alleged abuse). Do **NOT** list external cause codes
Terrorism	
Confirmed	FBI must identify event as act of terrorism. List first code Y38 (list more than one code if more than one act of terrorism). Then code for place of occurrence Y92.
Suspected	List code for assault. Do **NOT** list Y38 code
Secondary effects of terrorism	List first code for injury. List code Y38.9 for conditions occurring subsequent to terrorism event. Then list other Y38 codes if appropriate. Do **NOT** list this code for initial terrorist act.
Hurricane Victims - X37.0**	
Injury **directly** due to hurricane	Use as many external cause codes as needed to completely explain the circumstances: Codes for cause, intent, place, activity and status. List first code for hurricane. Examples: X37.0- Hurricane X30- Exposure to excessive natural heat X31- Exposure to excessive natural cold X38- Flood
Injury **indirectly** due to hurricane	List code for injury but **NOT** for hurricane (X37.0-.) Example: Patient injured in motor vehicle accident while evacuating due to incoming hurricane. Use external cause codes for motor vehicle accident, not hurricane.
Injury **may or may not** be due to hurricane	Assume the injury is due to the hurricane. Use code X37.0- and any appropriate external cause code(s).
Patient experienced hurricane but has **no injury**, adverse effect or poisoning as a result.	Do **NOT** list injury, external cause or Z codes.
Sequencing external causes	List hurricane code before other external cause codes except child and adult abuse and terrorism.
Treatment over multiple visits	Use external cause codes for each visit as appropriate. Use 7th digits A, D or S.
Documentation	Patient history may be very limited. Use any available documentation (not only from physician).

*Abuse includes: Bullying, intimidation, intimidation through social media, forced sexual exploitation, and forced labor exploitation.

Do **NOT code X36.0 (collapse of dam or man-made structure) for injuries due to hurricanes. This code is only used for collapse due to earth surface movements, not collapse due to hurricane.

Code also Z codes (Factors Influencing Health Status and Contact with Health Services) as appropriate. Examples are: homelessness or unavailability and inaccessibility of health-care facilities.

PART 4
Finding External Cause Codes –
Which, What, How, Who, When and Where

External cause codes include codes for:
- Activity Y93
- Place of occurrence Y92
- Patient status Y99
- Intent/cause of injury
    - Injuries due to accidents V00-V99
    - Injuries due to nonaccidents X71-Y35, Y38
    - Injuries related to military service Y36-Y37
    - Injuries related to medical treatment/complication Y62-Y84

Often activity, place of occurrence, and patient status are represented by digits within an intent/cause of injury code. For example:
V30.0XXA – Driver of three-wheeled motor vehicle injured in collision with pedestrian or animal in nontraffic accident.
- Activity – riding in three-wheeled motor vehicle
- Place of occurrence – nontraffic
- Patient status – driver

Additional codes might be added if appropriate to provide additional information. For example:
- Was the driver delivering goods for pay?
- Was the nontraffic place of occurrence a driveway or private road?

External cause codes can be divided into 4 different categories, each with subcategories. These are:

Categories of External Causes
Intent/Cause of Injury

Category - Accidents Subcategories - • Transport accidents • Other accidents	**Category - Military** Subcategories - • Military Operations • War Operations
Category - Nonaccidents Subcategories - • Assault • Self-harm • Legal intervention • Terrorism • Undetermined	**Category - Medical treatment** Subcategories - • Abnormal reactions to treatment • Adverse incidents due to medical devices • Complications • Misadventures

On the following page is a list of questions to ask when looking to code for external causes. It is suggested that the coder write these questions in their code book. The coder can then go down the list to ensure that all possible codes are selected.

This is followed by specific, step-by-step instructions on finding external cause codes in each category and subcategory.

Finding External Cause Codes – Which, What, Who, When, Where

Questions to Ask	Examples	
1. WHICH category/subcategory of external cause should be used?	Accidents Nonaccidents	Military Medical Treatment/complication
2. WHAT happened?	**Accidents –** Bite Cut Slipping Struck by/Striking against **Nonaccidents –** Legal intervention Self-harm Assault	**Military –** War operations Military operations **Medical treatment/ complications –** Abnormal reaction to medical treatment Adverse reaction to devices Misadventures
3. WHAT was the patient doing at the time of the injury?	What the patient was doing at the time of the injury: Cooking a meal Driving Jogging Painting a house Playing piano Playing soccer Working in an office	
4. WHO was the patient?	In most cases, use separate codes to indicate patient was employee, military on-duty, volunteer, etc. at time of injury	
	In these categories, digits within codes indicate who the patient was: Legal intervention (digits for bystander, law enforcement, suspect) Military (digits for civilian or military personnel) Terrorism (digits for civilian or public safety officer) Transport accidents (digits for driver, passenger, or hanger-on)	
5. WHEN was treatment given?	Initial encounter - A Subsequent encounter - D Sequelae – S	
6. WHERE was the patient when he/she was injured?	At residence, at work, in a park, in a store, in a public building, on a highway	

NOTES:
- Code first injury/condition from Alphabetic Index.
- Not all categories of external causes will include answers to all 6 of these questions.
- Not all categories of external causes will answer the questions in this order.
- Activity (WHAT was the patient doing?), Status of external cause (WHO was the patient?) and Place of occurrence (WHERE was the patient?) are listed only for initial visit.

CATEGORY OF INTENT/CAUSE - ACCIDENTS
Subcategories - Transport Accidents
Pedestrian & Pedestrian Conveyances
(Except for pedal cycle accidents) – Categories V00-V09

Questions	Digits	Examples
1. WHAT was the patient doing?	V00-V09	Patient was walking when they collided with: • Conveyance • Other pedestrian • Vehicle Patient was using conveyance when they collided with: • Other conveyance • Pedestrian • Vehicle
2. WHERE was the patient?	4th	In traffic, nontraffic or unspecified
3. WHAT happened?	4th	Patient on foot or On general type of conveyance (rolling-type, gliding-type, flat-bottomed)
	5th	Patient was on foot or On specific type of conveyance (roller-skates, skateboard, hoverboard, Segway).
	6th	In most cases, 6th digit indicates specific type of accident (fall, collided with, other accident). If no 6th digit, use 6th digit X.
4. WHEN was treatment given?	7th	A - Initial encounter D - Subsequent encounter S – Sequelae

List first code for injury/condition from Alphabetic Index.

For initial visit only, add these codes if the information is documented and codes will provide more information.
- WHO was the patient? Patient may be professional ice skater, skating instructor, sledding for leisure. Look under Status of external cause (Y99) in External Cause Index.
- WHERE was the patient when the injury occurred? Look under Place of occurrence (Y92) in External Cause index.

Examples pedestrian and pedestrian conveyances:
1. Anoxic brain damage due to previous head injury, three years ago, when patient was in traffic accident (struck by car) while walking along a highway.
   - Injury (anoxic brain damage) - G93.1
   - Pedestrian (on foot collided with car) (sequela) V03.10XS
   - Note: Activity, External cause status and Place of occurrence codes are not used for subsequent encounters.

Pedestrian & Pedestrian Conveyance (continued)

2. Patient fell off skateboard while on the sidewalk, resulting in lacerations on right knee. Initial encounter.
   - Injury (laceration of right knee) - S81.011A
   - Pedestrian conveyance (skateboard) (fall) - V00.131A
   - Status of external cause (leisure activity) – Y99.8
   - Place of occurrence (sidewalk) - Y92.480
   - Note: Activity code is not used since it would not add information.

3. Patient collided with pedestrian while sledding at a local middle school. Patient strained lower back. Initial encounter.
   - Injury (lower back) – S39.012A
   - Pedestrian conveyance (sled) - V00.228A
   - Status of external cause (leisure activity) – Y99.8
   - Place of occurrence (middle school) - Y92.212
   - Note: Activity code is not used since it would not add information.

CATEGORY OF INTENT/CAUSE - ACCIDENTS
Subcategories - Transport Accidents
Pedal Cyclist – Categories V10-V19

Questions	Digits	Examples
1. WHAT happened?	1st – 3rd	Pedal cyclist Noncollision or collision accident
	5th	In most cases, 5th digit is X. For V19 only – 5th digit for collision with unspecified or other specified vehicle
	6th	Use 6th digit X.
2. WHO was the patient?	4th	Driver Passenger Person boarding or alighting
3. WHERE was the patient?	4th	Traffic or nontraffic
4. WHEN was treatment given?	7th	A - Initial encounter D - Subsequent encounter S – Sequelae

List first code for injury/condition from Alphabetic Index.

For initial visit only, add these codes if the information is documented and codes will provide more information.
- WHAT was the patient doing? Look under Activity (Y93) in External Cause Index.
- WHO was the patient? Patient may be bicycle messenger or riding for leisure. Look under Status of external cause (Y99) in External Cause Index.
- WHERE was the patient when injury occurred? Patient may be on city street or in a park. Look under Place of occurrence (Y92) in External Cause index.

Examples Pedal cyclist:
1. Patient on bicycle (driver) was hit by a pick-up truck, resulting in a closed fracture, right foot. She was working as a messenger for a delivery service. Initial encounter. The patient was riding in a public parking lot at the time of the accident.
    - Injury (fracture) – S92.901A
    - Transport accident (bicycle and pick-up truck, traffic) - V13.4XXA
    - Place of occurrence (parking lot) - Y92.481
    - Status of external cause (civilian employee) - Y99.0
    - Note: Activity code not used because it would not add any additional information.

Pedal cycle accidents (continued)

2. Patient fell from his bicycle due to a ruptured tire, resulting in contusions on the left elbow. He was working as a volunteer delivering food to homebound patients, initial encounter. The accident occurred on the private driveway of a single family home.
   - Injury (contusion) – S50.02xA
   - Transport accident (pedal cycle, noncollision, nontraffic) – V18.0XXA
   - Accident (explosion, bicycle tire) - W37.0XXA
   - Place of occurrence (private driveway) - Y92.014
   - Status of external cause (volunteer) - Y99.2
   - Note: Activity code not used because it would not add any additional information.

3. Patient received a laceration on his forehead when he collided with telephone pole while alighting a rickshaw while on vacation. The accident occurred on a city street.
   - Injury (lacerations) – S01.81XA
   - Transport accident (pedal cycle, collision, stationary object, while alighting) – V17.3XXA
   - Place of occurrence (public street) – Y92.414
   - Status of external cause (leisure activity) – Y99.8

CATEGORY OF INTENT/CAUSE - ACCIDENTS
Subcategories - Transport Accidents
Other Land Vehicles V20-V89

Question	Digits	Examples
1. WHAT was the patient doing?	V20-V89	Patient riding in vehicle (car, motor cycle, bus, etc.)
2. WHAT happened?	V20-V89	Patient's vehicle and other vehicle collided or Patient's vehicle involved in noncollision accident. Other vehicle involved (not patient's vehicle) (car, motor cycle, bus, etc.)
	5th	In most cases, 5th digit is X. Used only for other vehicle involved, other and unspecified vehicles
	6th	In most cases, 6th digit is X. Some codes in category V80 (animal rider, animal drawn vehicle) include 6th digit with more specific information
3. WHO was the patient?	4th	Driver, passenger, unspecified, boarding or alighting
4. WHERE was the patient?	4th	Nontraffic or traffic
5. WHEN was treatment given?	7th	A - Initial encounter D - Subsequent encounter S – Sequelae

List first code for injury/condition from Alphabetic Index.

For initial visit only, add these codes if the information is documented and codes will provide more information.
- WHO was the patient? Look under Status of external cause (Y99) in External Cause Index.
- WHERE was the patient when injury occurred? Look under Place of occurrence (Y92) in External Cause index.

Do **NOT** use WHERE codes from category Y92.81- for type of vehicle.

Examples other land vehicles:
1. Deliveryman sprained his left ankle when he got off of a moving pick-up truck in a parking lot. Initial encounter.
   - Injury (sprain) – S93.402A
   - Transport accident (while alighting from pick-up truck) - V58.4XXA
   - Place of occurrence (parking lot) – Y92.481
   - Status of external cause (civilian working) – Y99.0

2. Military police officer received multiple facial lacerations while driving an automobile while on duty. He was in a collision with another (civilian) automobile on freeway, initial encounter.
   - Injury (lacerations) – S01.81XA
   - Transport accident (military car collided with civilian car) V86.04XA
   - Place of occurrence (freeway) – Y92.411
   - Status of external cause (military on duty) - Y99.1

Examples other land vehicles (continued):

3. Bus driver hit a bicyclist. The airbag went off, causing contusions of the driver's right chest area. The bus was on a state road at the time of the accident. Initial encounter.
    a. Injury (contusions) S20.211A
    b. Transport accident (bus collided with bicyclist) – V71.5XXA
    c. Accident (struck by, air bag) – W22.11XA
    d. Place of occurrence (state road) – Y92.413
    e. Status of external cause (civilian employee) – Y99.0

CATEGORY OF INTENT/CAUSE - ACCIDENTS
Subcategories - Transport Accidents
Water Accidents – V90-V94

Question	Digits	Examples
1. WHAT happened?	V90-V94	Drowning and submersion Other injury on watercraft Other and unspecified water transport accidents
	4th	More specific information Drowning and submersion due to watercraft – • Overturning • Sinking • Burning (patient fell or jumped off) • Crushed (patient fell or jumped off) Collision with another watercraft. Patient injured by - • Being crushed between 2 watercraft • Fall Patient onboard watercraft. Patient injured by - • Burn – watercraft on fire • Heat exposure • Fall • Struck by object • Explosion • Machinery accident Other injuries. Patient – • Was thrown/washed overboard due to motion of water • Fell from watercraft, hit object or bottom of body of water • Was bather (swimmer) struck by watercraft • Was rider of inflatable watercraft being pulled behind other watercraft • Was barefoot water-skier
2. WHAT was the patient doing?	5th	Patient riding on/in - Merchant ship Passenger ship Fishing board Sailboat Canoe or kayak Inflatable craft Powered or unpowered Water skis Watercraft being pulled
3. WHO was the patient?	6th	In most cases, 6th digit is X. For category V94.8- (other and unspecified accident) only – Patient was civilian on military watercraft
4. WHEN was treatment given?	7th	A - Initial encounter D - Subsequent encounter S – Sequelae

List first code for injury/condition from Alphabetic Index.

For initial visit only, add these codes if information is documented and codes will provide more information.
- WHAT was the patient doing? Look up Activity (Y93) in External Cause Index.
- WHO was the patient? Look under Status of external cause (Y99) in External Cause Index.
- WHERE was the patient when injury occurred? Look under Place of occurrence (Y92) in External Cause index (river or lake).

Do **NOT** use WHERE codes from category Y92.8- for type of watercraft.

Examples water transport:

1. Patient was nearly drowned when her luxury cruise ship sank in a harbor off Fort Lauderdale. The patient was the ship's cook and was preparing breakfast at the time. Initial encounter.
    - Injury (near drowning) – T75.1XXA
    - Transport accident (watercraft, passenger ship, sank) – V90.11XA
    - Activity (cooking) - Y93.G3
    - Place of occurrence (harbor) – Y92.89
    - Status of external cause (civilian employee) – Y99.0

2. Patient was swimming with friends in a river when he was hit by a ferry boat. He suffered an open wound of the left shoulder. Initial encounter.
    - Injury (open wound) – S41.002A
    - Transport accident (watercraft, swimmer hit by powered boat) – Y94.11XA
    - Place of occurrence (river) – Y92.828
    - Status of external cause (leisure activity) – Y99.8
    - Note: No activity code is used because it would not add additional information.

3. Patient's chest was crushed when he was caught between two kayaks while on vacation. Accident occurred on a lake.
    - Injury (crush injury, chest) – S28.0XXA
    - Transport accident (watercraft, kayaks, crush injury) – V91.15XA
    - Place of occurrence (lake) – Y92.828
    - Status of external cause (leisure activity) – Y99.8

CATEGORY OF INTENT/CAUSE - ACCIDENTS
Subcategories - Transport Accidents
Air and Space Transport Accidents – V95-V97

Question	Digits	Examples
1. WHAT was the patient doing?	V95-V97	General type of vehicle involved patient was in/on Powered aircraft, nonpowered aircraft or Other specified
	4th	Specific vehicle patient was in/on (helicopter, balloon, commercial airplane, spaceship) Person on ground injured by aircraft
2. WHAT happened?	5th	Crash, collision, forced landing, fire, explosion
3. WHO was the patient?	6th	In most cases, 6th digit is X. For category V97.8- (other and unspecified accident) only – Patient was civilian on military watercraft or patient on ground who was injured by aircraft
4. WHEN was treatment given?	7th	A - Initial encounter D - Subsequent encounter S – Sequelae

List first code for injury/condition from Alphabetic Index.

For initial visit only, add this code if the information is documented and code will provide more information.
- WHO was the patient? Look under Status of external cause (Y99) in External Cause Index.

Do **NOT** use these codes for military aircraft accidents occurring during military or war operations. See categories Y36-Y37

Do **NOT** use WHERE place of occurrence code Y92.8- for type of aircraft.

Do **NOT** use these codes for military aircraft accidents in military or war operations. See categories Y36-Y37

Examples AIR transport:
1. Patient, working as a maid, was in the kitchen of a house when it was hit by a small plane. She was mopping the floor at the time of the accident. She suffered minor cuts and bruises to the lower back.
    - Injury (cuts and bruises) – S30.91XA
    - Transport accident (airplane, patient on ground) – V97.31XA
    - Activity (mopping) – Y93.E5
    - Place of occurrence (kitchen of single family house) – Y92.010
    - Status of external cause (employed civilian) – Y99.0

Examples AIR/SPACE transport (continued):

2. Patient was a passenger in a hot air balloon when he was injured when the balloon hit some power lines. The patient suffered some second degree electrical burns on his hands. Initial encounter.
   - Injury (electrical burns) – T23.202A (left hand), T23.201A (right hand)
   - Transport accident (hot air balloon, passenger) – V96.03XA
   - Status of external cause (leisure activity) -Y99.8
   - Note: No activity or place of occurrence code is used.

3. Patient was copilot of airplane when he fell in the aisle on the way to the bathroom. He dislocated his right hip in the fall.
   - Injury (dislocated hip) – S73.004A
   - Transport accident (fall in, on, or from aircraft) – V97.0XXA
   - Status of external cause (employed civilian) – Y99.0
   - Note: No activity or place of occurrence codes used because they would not add any information.

CATEGORY OF INTENT/CAUSE - ACCIDENTS
Subcategory - Other Accidental Injuries W00-X58

Question	Digits	Examples
1. WHAT happened?	W00-X58	Slipping, tripping, stumbling falls W00-W19 Exposure to inanimate mechanical forces W20-W49 Exposure to animate mechanical forces W50-W64 Drowning and submersion W65-W74 Electrical current, radiation and extreme air temperature/pressure W85-W99 Exposure to smoke, fire and flames X00-X08 Contact with heat and hot substances X10-X19 Exposure to forces of nature X30-X39 Overexertion and strenuous or repetitive movements X50 Other specified factors X52-X58
	4th	Used for most but not all categories. If no 4th digit, use 4th digit X Provide more specific information such as: Specific type of firearm Fell from or into specific place Jumped from specific place Slipped without falling Struck by specific object Bitten by dog
	5th	For some categories, use 5th digit X. For other categories, digit provides additional information. For example, code W61.33-, pecked by chicken.
	6th	For some categories, use 6th digit X. Other categories, digit provides additional information For example, code W34.111-, accidental malfunction of paintball gun.
2. WHEN was treatment given?	7th	A - Initial encounter D - Subsequent encounter S – Sequelae

List first code for injury/condition from Alphabetic Index.

For initial visit only, add these codes if the information is documented and codes will provide more information.
- WHAT was the patient doing? Look up Activity (Y93) in External Cause Index.
- WHO was the patient? Look under Status of external cause (Y99) in External Cause Index.
- WHERE was the patient when injury occurred? Look under Place of occurrence (Y92) in External Cause index.

Examples other accidents:

1. Patient bitten by stray dog, causing lacerations on his right lower leg. Patient was at an amusement park with his son at the time of the accident.
   - Injury (lacerations) - S81.811A
   - Accident (contact with, animal, dog, bite) - W54.0XXA
   - Place of occurrence (amusement park) – Y92.831
   - Status of external cause (leisure) – Y99.8

2. Patient fell from a ladder while working inside a building construction site. Patient has superficial cuts and bruises on his left shoulder. Patient is an employed construction worker, initial encounter.
   - Injury (cuts and bruises) – S40.012A
   - Accident (fall, from ladder) – W11.XXxA
   - Activity (working in construction) Y93.H3
   - Place of occurrence (building under construction) – Y92.61
   - Status of external cause (civilian employee) Y99.0

3. Patient injured by rifle, which resulted in open wound in abdomen into peritoneal cavity. Accident occurred while patient was hunting in a forest with a group of friends.
   - Injury (abdominal wound) – S31.609A
   - Accident (discharge, hunting rifle) – W33.02XA
   - Place of occurrence (forest) – Y92.821
   - Status of external cause (leisure) – Y99.8
   - Note: No specific activity code for hunting

4. Patient suffered second degree burns of the thighs when she dropped a cup of hot coffee in her lap. She was at a fast-food restaurant having breakfast at the time.
   - Injury (burns to thighs) - T24.212A (left thigh), T24.211A (right thigh)
   - Accident (contact with, hot drinks) - X10.0XXA
   - Place of occurrence (restaurant) - Y92.511
   - Status of external cause (leisure) – Y99.8

5. Patient fell asleep on the sofa with a lit cigarette. He was in his apartment living room watching television. The sofa ignited and the patient suffered third degree burns to left forearm.
   - Injury (burns to arm) – T22.312A
   - Accident (exposure to, fire, flames, sofa fire, due to burning cigarette) – X08.11XA
   - Place of occurrence (apartment living room) – Y92.038
   - Status of external cause (leisure) – Y99.8

6. Patient jumped into public swimming pool and hit her head, striking against side wall of the pool. She suffered a concussion with loss of consciousness for 20 minutes.
   - Injury (concussion) – S06.0X1A
   - Accident (striking against, wall, swimming pool, diving or jumping into water) – W16.532A
   - Place of occurrence (swimming pool) – Y92.34
   - Status of external cause (leisure) – Y99.8

CATEGORY OF INTENT/CAUSE - NONACCIDENTS
Subcategory Assault X92-Y09*

Question	Digits	Examples
1. WHAT happened?	X92-Y09	Assault by drowning/submersion Assault by firearm Assault by explosive material Assault by smoke, fire and flames Assault by steam, hot vapors and hot objects Assault by sharp object Assault by blunt object Assault by pushing from high place Assault by pushing/placing victim in front of moving object Assault by pushing/placing victim in from of subway train Assault by crashing motor vehicle Assault by bodily force Assault, unspecified
	4th	More specific information – Type of assault by bodily force (human bite, unarmed brawl) Type of sharp object (knife, dagger, glass) Type of bomb (gasoline, pipe)
	5th	For most categories, use X for 5th digit. Exceptions: X95 (other and unspecified firearm/gun) Y08 (assault by sports equipment and other specific means)
	6th	Use 6th digit X.
2. WHEN was treatment given?	7th	A - Initial encounter D - Subsequent encounter S – Sequelae

Code first for injury from Alphabetic Index.
*See next page for discussion of category Y07 – Perpetrator of assault, maltreatment and neglect\

For initial visit only, use additional codes if the information is documented and codes will provide more information. For example:
- WHAT was the patient doing? Look up Activity (Y93) in External Cause Index.
- WHO is patient? Look under Status of external cause (Y99) in External Cause Index.
- WHERE did injury occur? Look under Place of occurrence (Y92) in External Cause index.

(continued on next page)

In the Assault subcategory, there are also codes for the perpetrator of assault, maltreatment and neglect. Use in addition to other external cause codes for confirmed assault if information is available.

Question	Digits	Examples
1. WHO victimized the patient?	Y09	Perpetrator of assault, maltreatment and neglect
	4th	Spouse or partner, parent, other family member Non-family member
	5th	More specific information – Sibling Husband Friend of parent Wife Daycare provider
	6th	Most codes use 6th digit X. Exception: Y07.4- and Y07.5-
2. WHEN was treatment given?	7th	A - Initial encounter D - Subsequent encounter S – Sequelae

Examples assault:

1. Patient injured when he was assaulted with a baseball bat in public parking garage, initial encounter. Patient has concussion but did not lose consciousness.
   - Injury (concussion, no loss of consciousness) - S06.0X0A
   - Assault (struck by, sports equipment, baseball bat) - Y08.02XA
   - Place of occurrence (parking garage) - Y92.481
   - Notes: No information concerning patient status or activity

2. Patient injured during a suspected terrorist attack. The FBI has not confirmed that this was terrorism. The patient was in a downtown street when he was hit by a speeding car. Patient was working at a food cart at the time. The patient received multiple fractured ribs on the right and left sides. Initial encounter.
   - Injury (fractured ribs) - S22.43XA
   - Assault (This is coded as an assault since terrorism was not confirmed by the FBI.) - Y03.0XXA
   - Place of occurrence (downtown street) - Y92.414
   - Patient status (working for pay) – Y99.0

3. This woman was injured when she was assaulted by her husband. She presented with lacerations of the face. He had attacked her with a knife. Initial encounter.
   - Injury (lacerations) – S01.81
   - Assault (knife) – X99.1
   - Perpetrator (husband) – Y07.01
   - Notes: No information concerning patient status or activity.

CATEGORY OF INTENT/CAUSE - NONACCIDENTS
Subcategory - Intentional Self-Harm* X71-X83

Question	Digits	Examples
1. WHAT happened?	X71-X83	Self-harm by drowning/submersion Self-harm by firearm Self-harm by explosive material Self-harm by smoke, fire and flames Self-harm by steam, hot vapors and hot objects Self-harm by sharp object Self-harm by blunt object Self-harm by jumping from high place Self-harm by jumping/lying in front of moving object Self-harm by crashing motor vehicle Self-harm by other specified means
	4th	Some codes use 4th digit X. For other codes, digit provides additional information – Location of drowning/submersion (bathtub, swimming pool) Type of firearm (shotgun, machine gun) Type of sharp object (knife, dagger, glass)
	5th	Most categories use 5th digit X. Exception: X74 (other and unspecified firearm and gun)
	6th	Use 6th digit X.
2. WHEN was treatment given?	7th	A - Initial encounter D - Subsequent encounter S – Sequelae

*Includes purposely self-inflicted injury and suicide attempts.

Code first for injury from Alphabetic Index.
For initial visit only, use additional codes if the information is documented and codes will provide more information. For example:
- WHAT was the patient doing? Look up Activity (Y93) in External Cause Index.
- WHO is patient? Look under Status of external cause (Y99) in External Cause Index.
- WHERE did injury occur? Look under Place of occurrence (Y92) in External Cause index.

Examples:
1. Patient in the bathroom of her hospital room attempted suicide by cutting her left wrist with a piece of glass.
    - Injury (laceration of wrist) – S61.512A
    - Attempted suicide (sharp glass) - X78.0XXA
    - Status of external cause (specified NEC-patient) - Y99.8
    - Place of occurrence (hospital bathroom) - Y92.231

2. Patient presented with fractures of lower ends of both femurs after falling/jumping from high building (a factory). The physician documented that he could not determine whether the injury was accidental, an assault, or a suicide attempt.
    - Injury (fractures) - S72.401A (right femur), S72.042A (left femur)
    - Undetermined intent (high building) - Y30.XXxA
    - Place of occurrence (factory) - Y92.63
    - Notes: No information concerning patient status or activity.

3. An elderly patient, living in her sister's mobile home, is seen with severe dehydration. The condition is confirmed abuse (neglect) by the sister.
    - Injury (neglect, confirmed) – T74.01XXA
    - Injury (dehydration) – E86.0
    - Perpetrator (sister) – Y07.411
    - Place of occurrence (mobile home) – Y92.029
    - Notes: No information concerning patient status or activity

CATEGORY OF INTENT/CAUSE - NONACCIDENTS
Subcategory - Legal Intervention Y35

Questions	Digits	Examples
1. WHAT happened?	Y35	Legal intervention
	4th	More specific information – Legal intervention involving firearm discharge Legal intervention involving explosives Legal intervention involving gas Legal intervention involving blunt object Legal intervention involving sharp object Legal intervention involving other specified means Legal intervention, unspecified
	5th	More specific information – Blunt object, baton Gas, tear gas Explosives, dynamite Sharp object, bayonet Firearm discharge, handgun Other means, manhandling
2. WHO is the patient?	6th	1 - Law enforcement officer (on or off duty) 2 – Bystander 3 - Suspect 9 – Unspecified
3. WHEN was treatment given?	7th	A - Initial encounter D - Subsequent encounter S – Sequelae

Code first for injury/condition using Alphabetic Index.
Additional codes – Use if information is available and only for initial visit
- WHAT was the patient doing? See Activity (Y93) (what bystander or officer were doing when injured)
- WHERE did the injury happen? See Place of occurrence (Y92)
- WHO (for civilian patient only). Example: civilian working for pay

Examples Legal Intervention:
1. Bank teller was injured during shootout between police officer and suspect. Injury was open wound in abdominal wall. The weapon was a handgun.
    - Injury (open wound in abdominal wall) – S31.109A
    - Legal intervention (injury to bystander) – Y35.022A
    - External cause status (civilian employee) – Y99.0
    - Place of occurrence (bank) – Y92.510
    - Note - No information on activity

2. Previous patient seen for follow-up visit.
    - Injury (open wound in abdominal wall) – S31.109D
    - Legal intervention (injury to bystander) – Y35.022D
    - Note - Activity, Status of external cause and Place of occurrence codes are not used for follow-up visits.

Examples Legal Intervention (continued):

3. Suspect in bank robbery was injured by police officer's use of a stun gun, resulting in second degree burn of the lower right arm. The injury occurred on the sidewalk outside the bank as the robber was trying to flee.
    - Injury (second degree burn) – T22.211A
    - Legal intervention (injury to suspect) – Y35.833A
    - Place of occurrence (sidewalk) – Y92.480
    - Note: Activity, Status of External Cause codes are not used.

CATEGORY OF INTENT/CAUSE - NONACCIDENTS
Subcategory Terrorism – Y38

Questions	Digits	Examples
	Y38	Terrorism
1. WHAT happened?	4th	More specific information – Terrorism involving explosion of marine weapons Terrorism involving destruction of aircraft Terrorism involving other explosions and fragments Terrorism involving fires, conflagration, and hot substances Terrorism involving firearms Terrorism involving nuclear weapons Terrorism involving biological weapons Terrorism involving chemical weapons Terrorism involving other and unspecified means Terrorism, secondary effects
	5th	Most categories use 5th digit X. Exception: Y38.8- (Terrorism involving other and unspecified means, including suicide bomber)
2. WHO was the patient?	6th	1 - Public safety officer 2 – Civilian 3 – Terrorist
3. WHEN was treatment given?	7th	A - Initial encounter D - Subsequent encounter S – Sequelae

List first code for injury/condition from Alphabetic Index.

For initial visit only, add these codes if the information is documented and codes will provide more information.
- WHAT was the patient doing? Look under Activity (Y93) in External Cause Index.
- WHO was the patient? Use for civilian (6th digit 2) only. If additional information available, look under status of external cause (Y99) in External Cause Index.
- WHERE was the patient when injury occurred? Look under Place of occurrence (Y92) in External Cause index.

Examples Terrorism:
1. Civilian, running for exercise on the sidewalk, was injured due to destruction of aircraft (explosion), confirmed by FBI as terrorist attack. Patient inhaled unspecified toxic fumes.
   - Injury (inhalation of toxic fumes) (use 5th digit for assault) - T59.93XA
   - Terrorism (injury due to destruction of aircraft) (injury to civilian) - Y38.1X2A
   - Activity (running) - Y93.02
   - External cause status (leisure activity) – Y99.8
   - Place of occurrence (sidewalk) - Y92.480

2. On-duty police officer received skull fracture in courthouse destroyed by terrorist bomb.
   - Injury (unspecified skull fracture) - S02.91XA
   - Terrorism (public safety officer) (injury due to bomb) - Y38.2X1A
   - Place of occurrence (courthouse) – Y92.240
   - Note: Activity, Status of external cause codes are not used.

Examples, terrorism (continued)

3. A terrorist was detained after he used a car to run down civilians in a public park. He had an open wound in his left thigh after being shot by a police officer using a handgun.
    - Injury (open wound in left thigh) - S71.102A
    - Terrorism (injury due to firearm) (injury to terrorist) – Y38.4X3A
    - Place of occurrence (public park) – Y92.830
    - Note: Activity, Status of external cause codes are not used.

CATEGORY OF INTENT/CAUSE - NONACCIDENTS
Subcategory Undetermined

Questions	Digits	Examples
1. WHAT happened?	Y21-Y33	General type of event. Undetermined intent, drowning and submersion Undetermined intent, firearm discharge Undetermined intent, explosive material Undetermined intent, smoke, fire and flames Undetermined intent, hot vapors and hot objects Undetermined intent, sharp object Undetermined intent, blunt object Undetermined intent, falling/jumping/pushed from high place Undetermined intent, falling/lying/running before or into moving object Undetermined intent, crashing motor vehicle Undetermined intent, other specified events
	4th	Some categories use 4th digit X. For other codes, digit provides additional information, such as: Location of drowning/submersion (bathtub, swimming pool) Type of firearm (shotgun, machine gun) Type of sharp object (knife, dagger, glass)
	5th	Use 5th digit X.
	6th	Use 6th digit X.
2. WHEN was treatment given?	7th	A - Initial encounter D - Subsequent encounter S – Sequelae

List first code for injury/condition from Alphabetic Index.

For initial visit only, add these codes if the information is documented and codes will provide more information.
- WHAT was the patient doing? Look under Activity (Y93) in External Cause Index.
- WHO was the patient? Use for civilian (6th digit 2) only. If additional information available, look under status of external cause (Y99) in External Cause Index.
- WHERE was the patient when injury occurred? Look under Place of occurrence (Y92) in External Cause index.

Examples Undetermined intent:

1. Patient presented with laceration of the right forearm caused by a piece of glass. The physician documented that he could not determine whether the injury was due to an accident, assault, self-harm or other cause.
   - Injury (cut by glass) - S51.811A
   - Undetermined intent - V28.0-

2. Patient almost drowned in the family swimming pool in her backyard. The physician documented that she could not determine whether the injury was due to an accident, assault, self-harm or other cause. Subsequent encounter.
   - Injury (near drowning) – T75.1XXD
   - Undetermined intent – V21.2XXD
   - Note: Activity, Patient Status and Place of Occurrence codes are not used for subsequent visits.

CATEGORY OF INTENT/CAUSE - MILITARY
Subcategory Military Operations– Y37

Questions	Digits	Examples
1. WHAT happened?	Y37	Military operations
	4th	General category – Military operations involving explosion of maritime weapons Military operations involving destruction of aircraft Military operations involving other explosives and fragments Military operations involving fires, conflagrations and hot substances Military operations involving firearm discharge/other forms of conventional warfare Military operations involving nuclear weapons Military operations involving biological weapons Military operations involving chemical weapons or other forms of unconventional warfare Military operations involving other and unspecified means
	5th	More specific information – Explosion of maritime weapons, involving depth-charge Destruction of aircraft, due to collision with other aircraft Other explosives and fragments, aerial bomb Fires, conflagrations and hot substances, gasoline bomb Firearm discharge/other forms of conventional warfare, rubber bullets Nuclear weapons, direct blast effect Other and unspecified, friendly fire
2. WHO was the patient?	6th	0 - Military personnel 1- Civilian working with military
3. WHEN was treatment given?	7th	A - Initial encounter D - Subsequent encounter S – Sequelae

List first code for injury/condition from Alphabetic Index.

For initial visit only, add these codes if the information is documented and codes will provide more information.
- WHAT was the patient doing? Patient may have been marching, rock climbing, or SCUBA diving. Look under Activity (Y93) in External Cause Index.
- WHERE was the patient when injury occurred? Look under Place of occurrence (Y92) in External Cause index.

Do **NOT** use these codes if patient is a member of the military but is not in a war environment or on military property at the time of injury. Use codes from other categories (such as accident or assault) with WHO patient status code for military - Y99.1 or Y99.8.

Do **NOT** use these codes if injury resulted from military transport accident with civilian vehicle. Use codes from Transport accidents V00-V94 with 4th and 5th digits 81.

Examples: Military Operations

1. Army private injured by an IED (improvised explosive device) which exploded accidentally on a military base in California. The injury resulted in a primary blast injury of both ears. Initial encounter.
    - Injury (blast injury to ears) - S09.313A.
    - Military (IED, injury to military personnel) Y37.260A
    - Place of occurrence (military base) - Y92.139
    - Note: Activity and Status codes are not used since they would not add new information.

2. Civilian patient was working as a consultant on a military training ground in Missouri. He was injured when he came too close to a flamethrower. Initial encounter.
    - Military (flamethrower, civilian) - Y37.321A
    - Place of occurrence (military training ground) – Y92.84
    - Patient status (working for salary) – Y99.0
    - Note: Activity code not used since it would not add new information.

CATEGORY OF INTENT/CAUSE - MILITARY
Subcategory Operations of War - Y36

Questions	Digits	Examples
1. WHAT happened?	Y36	Operations of war
	4th	More specific information – Operations of war involving explosion of maritime weapons Operations of war involving destruction of aircraft Operations of war involving other explosives and fragments Operations of war involving fires, conflagrations and hot substances Operations of war involving firearm discharge/other forms of conventional warfare Operations of war involving nuclear weapons Operations of war involving biological weapons Operations of war involving chemical weapons or other forms of unconventional warfare Operations of war after cessation of hostilities Operations of war involving other and unspecified means
	5th	More specific information – Explosion of maritime weapons, involving depth-charge Destruction of aircraft, due to collision with other aircraft Other explosives and fragments, aerial bomb Fires, conflagrations and hot substances, gasoline bomb Firearm discharge/other forms of conventional warfare, rubber bullets Nuclear weapons, direct blast effect Other and unspecified, friendly fire
2. WHO was the patient?	6th	0 - Military personnel 1 - Civilian working with military
3. WHEN was treatment given?	7th	A - Initial encounter D - Subsequent encounter S – Sequelae

List first code for injury/condition from Alphabetic Index.

For initial visit only, add these codes if the information is documented and codes will provide more information.
- WHAT was the patient doing? Patient may have been marching, rock climbing, or SCUBA diving. Look under Activity (Y93) in External Cause Index.
- WHERE was the patient when injury occurred? Look under Place of occurrence (Y92) in External Cause index.

Do **NOT** use these codes if patient is a member of the military but is not in a war environment or on military property at the time of injury. Use codes from other categories (such as accident or assault) with WHO patient status code for military - Y99.1 or Y99.8.

Do **NOT** use these codes if injury resulted from military transport accident with civilian vehicle. Use codes from Transport accidents V00-V94 with 4th and 5th digits 81.

Examples Operations of War:

1. Navy officer injured by chemical weapon burns to face while in Iraqi desert. He is now seen in hospital in Baltimore for continued care.
    - Injury (chemical burn on face) - T20.00XD
    - War operations (chemical weapon burn, injury to military personnel) - Y36.7X0D
    - Status and place of occurrence codes are not used for subsequent care

2. New York Times reporter, imbedded with army platoon in Iraq, was injured by gasoline bomb. Patient has burns over 50% of his body, 22% third degree burns. Initial encounter.
    - Injury (burns) – T31.52
    - War operations (gasoline bomb, injury to civilian personnel) – Y36.311A
    - Place of occurrence (desert) – Y92.820
    - Status of external cause (civilian employee) – Y99.0
    - Note: Activity code not used since it would not add new information.

CATEGORY – MEDICAL TREATMENT/COMPLICATION
Subcategory – Misadventure Y62-Y69

Question	Digits	Examples
1. WHAT happened?	Y62-Y69	Misadventure involving failure of sterile precautions Misadventure involving failure in dosage Misadventure involving contaminated medical/biological substances Misadventure involving nonadministration of surgical/medical care Misadventures, other specified
	4th	More specific information – Specific failure (such as sterile precautions, during dialysis) Specific surgery/procedure (such as transplants, catheterization) Method used to introduce medical or biological substance Wrong procedure/wrong patient
	5th	Most codes use 5th digit X. Exception: Subcategory Y65.5- (performance of wrong procedure) Include 5th digits for wrong patient or wrong procedure.

NOTES: These codes use 4 or 5 digits only. Do NOT use 6th or 7th digits.
Do **NOT** use additional codes for WHAT was the patient doing, WHERE the injury occurred or WHO is the patient with these codes.

Examples misadventures:

1. Patient received transfusion of substance which was contaminated with bacteria. As a result, the patient developed sepsis.
    - Injury (transfusion leading to infection) – T80.22XA (plus codes for infectious agent if known)
    - Injury (sepsis) – A41.9
    - Misadventure (contaminated substance transfused) – Y64.0

2. Patient was seen for hernia surgery. Due to a mix-up in the medical records, the physician performed an appendectomy instead.
    - Injury (complication of digestive surgery) K91.81 (plus code for reason for hernia surgery)
    - Misadventure (wrong procedure) Y65.51

CATEGORY – MEDICAL TREATMENT/COMPLICATION
Subcategory – Injuries Related to Adverse Reaction to Medical Devices Y70-82

Question	Digits	Examples
1. WHAT happened?	Y70-Y82	Adverse reaction to medical devices listed by: • Medical specialty (such as anesthesiology) • Body system (such as cardiovascular, ophthalmic) • General hospital and personal-use devices • Other and unspecified devices
	4th	Purpose of medical device: • Diagnostic and monitoring • Therapeutic and rehabilitative • Prosthetic or • Other implants, surgical instruments, miscellaneous
	5th	Most codes use 5th digit X. Exception: Y7.1- (specific ophthalmic device)

NOTES: These codes use 4 or 5 digits only. They do NOT add 6th or 7th digits.

Do **NOT** use additional codes for WHAT was the patient doing, WHERE the injury occurred or WHO is the patient with these codes.

CATEGORY – MEDICAL TREATMENT/COMPLICATION
Subcategory - Injuries Related to Abnormal Reaction to Medical Treatment Y83-Y84

Question	Digits	Examples
1. WHAT happened?	Y83-Y84	Abnormal reaction to surgical operation/other surgical procedures Abnormal reaction to other medical procedures, or later complication, without mention of misadventure at time of procedure
	4th	Y83 – Lists surgical procedures, such as: • Transplant of whole organ (organ not specified) • Implant of artificial internal device (device not specified) • Anastomosis, bypass or graft (no additional information) • Formation of stoma (organ/location not specified) • Other reconstructive surgery Y84- List medical procedures, such as: • Cardiac catheterization • Kidney dialysis • Radiological procedure/radiotherapy • Shock therapy • Aspiration of fluid • Insertion of gastric or duodenal sound • Urinary catheterization • Blood sampling • Other and unspecified

NOTES: These codes use 4 digits only. Do NOT add 5-7th digits.

Do **NOT** use additional codes for WHAT was the patient doing, WHERE the injury occurred or WHO is the patient with these codes.

Sometimes multiple codes are needed to completely describe the circumstances. These are identified by the use of Excludes2 notes. Some of these categories also have Excludes1 notes. For example:

Code Category	Excludes2 Notes Code also if appropriate -	Excludes1 Notes Do NOT code also -
Y62-Y65 Misadventure	Breakdown or malfunction of device Y70-Y82	Abnormal reaction or later complication Y83-Y84
Y70-Y82 Adverse incidents involving device	Later complications without breakdown or malfunction of device Y83-Y84 Misadventures Y62-Y69 Abnormal reaction to treatment Y83-Y84	No codes listed
Y83-Y84 Abnormal reaction to treatment	Breakdown or malfunction of device Y70-Y82	Misadventures Y62-Y65

Examples: Medical Treatment/Complications

1. Patient had inflammatory response to presence of pacemaker. Device is functioning properly.
   - Injury (reaction to pacemaker) T82.7XXA (plus code for reason for pacemaker insertion)
   - Abnormal reaction to implant of internal device (pacemaker) Y83.1
   - Adverse incident, therapeutic cardiovascular device (complication of surgery to insert pacemaker) - Y71.1

2. Patient has hernia surgery last month but now the mesh used in the surgery is displaced.
   - Injury (displaced implant, gastrointestinal device) (the mesh) - T85.528A
   - Adverse incident (gastroenterology and urology device, prosthetic and implants) Y73.2
   - Complication (complication, surgical procedure, anastomosis, bypass or graft) Y83.2

3. Patient suffered breakdown of catheter during dialysis procedure.
   - Injury (mechanical complication of catheter) T82.41xA
   - Adverse incident (gastroenterology and urology device, therapeutic device) Y73.1
   - Complication (complication, medical procedure, kidney dialysis) – Y84.1

Part 5 - Index of External Cause of Injuries

Introduction

Following is a simplified version of the official ICD-10-CM Index to External Causes.

The index has separate sections for these codes:
- Activity Y93
- Place of occurrence Y92
- Patient status Y99
- Intent/cause of injury
    - Injuries due to accidents V00-V99
        - Transport accidents (air/space, land, and water accidents)
        - Other accidents
    - Injuries due to nonaccidents X71-Y35, Y38 (assault, intentional self-harm, legal intervention, and terrorism)
    - Injuries related to military service Y36-Y37 (military operations and operations of war)
    - Injuries related to medical treatment/complication Y62-Y84 (misadventures, adverse reactions to devices, and abnormal reaction to medical treatment)
- Supplemental factors
- Sequelae coding

Notes: The term "pedestrian conveyance" is not used if a specific type of conveyance is documented (such as roller skates, wheelchair or skis). These pedestrian conveyances are listed alphabetically under their own entry. Specified and unspecified conveyances are listed under heading Pedestrian conveyance and then by type of conveyance (rolling, gliding or flat-bottomed).

See Part 3 of this book for definitions of terms used in the Index.

BE SURE TO CONFIRM CODE IN TABULAR LIST!

Activity – A TO D

ICD-10-CM External Cause of Injuries Index
ACTIVITY (what the patient doing or using at the time of the injury) Y93

A	
Aerobic and step exercise (class) Y93.A3	
	water aerobics Y93.14
Animal care NEC Y93.K9	
	grooming Y93.K3
	milking Y93.K2
	shearing Y93.K3
	walking Y93.K1
Arts and handcrafts NEC Y93.D9 - *see also* specific Activity	
Athletics NEC Y93.79 - *see also* specific sport	
	sport played as a team or group NEC Y93.69
	sport played individually NEC Y93.59
B	
Baking Y93.G3	
Ballet Y93.41	
Barbells Y93.B3	
BASE jumping (Building, Antenna, Span, Earth) Y93.33	
Baseball Y93.64	
Basketball Y93.67	
Bathing (personal) Y93.E1	
	another person Y93.F1
Beach volleyball Y93.68	
Bike riding Y93.55	
	stationary bike Y93.A1
Blackout game Y93.85	
Boogie boarding Y93.18	
Bowling Y93.54	
Boxing Y93.71	
Brass instrument playing Y93.J4	
Building construction Y93.H3	
Bungee jumping Y93.34	
C	
Calisthenics Y93.A2	
Canoeing Y93.16	
Capture the flag Y93.6A	
Cardiorespiratory exercise NEC Y93.A9	
Caregiving (providing) NEC Y93.F9	
	bathing (another person) Y93.F1
	lifting (another person) Y93.F2
Cellular (using) telephone and other handheld device	
	communication device Y93.C2
	telephone Y93.C2
Challenge course Y93.A5	
Cheerleading Y93.45	

C (continued)	
Choking game Y93.85	
Circuit training Y93.A4	
Cleaning	
	clothes Y93.E2
	floor Y93.E5
	vacuuming Y93.E3
Climbing NEC Y93.39 – *see also* Rappelling and Jumping	
	mountain Y93.31
	rock Y93.31
	wall Y93.31
Combatives (martial arts) Y93.75	
Computer – *see also* Electronic (games) and Cellular	
	keyboarding Y93.C1
	technology NEC Y93.C9
Confidence course Y93.A5	
Construction (building) Y93.H3	
Cooking and baking Y93.G3	
Cool down exercises Y93.A2	
Cricket Y93.69	
Crocheting Y93.D1	
Cross country skiing Y93.24	
D	
Dancing (all types) Y93.41	
Digging (dirt) Y93.H1	
Dishwashing Y93.G1	
Diving (platform) (springboard) Y93.12	
	underwater Y93.15
Dodge ball Y93.6A	
Downhill skiing Y93.23	
Drum playing Y93.J2	
Dumbbells Y93.B3	

Note: Do **NOT** use activity codes for poisoning, adverse effects, underdosing, misadventures, sequelae or toxic effects.

Activity Codes – E to L

ACTIVITY Codes Y93

E

Electronic (games)
- devices NEC Y93.C9
- hand held interactive Y93.C2
- game playing (using) (with) keyboard or other stationary device Y93.C1

Elliptical machine Y93.A1

Exercise(s) (using machines) - *see also* specific exercise or machine
- cardiorespiratory conditioning Y93.A1
- muscle strengthening Y93.B1
  - non-machine NEC Y93.B9
- warm up or cool down exercises Y93.A2

External motion NEC Y93.I9
- roller coaster Y93.I1

F

Fainting game Y93.85
Field hockey Y93.65
Figure skating (pairs) (singles) Y93.21
Floor mopping and cleaning Y93.E5
Food Y93.G9
- cooking and baking Y93.G3
- grilling and smoking Y93.G2
- preparation and clean up 93.G1

Football (American) NOS Y93.61
- flag Y93.62
- tackle Y93.61
- touch Y93.62

Four square game Y93.6A
Free weights Y93.B3
Frisbee (ultimate) Y93.74
Furniture
- building Y93.D3
- finishing Y93.D3
- repair Y93.D3

G

Game playing (electronic) – *see* Electronic (games)
Gardening Y93.H2
Golf Y93.52
Grass drills Y93.A6
Grilling and smoking food Y93.G2
Grooming and shearing an animal Y93.K3
Guerilla drills Y93.A6
Gymnastics (rhythmic) Y93.42

H

Handball Y93.73
Handcrafts NEC Y93.D9 – *see also* specific craft
Hand held interactive device Y93.C2
Hang gliding Y93.35
Hiking (on level or elevated terrain) Y93.01
Hockey (ice) Y93.22
- field Y93.65

Horseback riding Y93.52
Horseplay Y93.83
Household maintenance – *see* specific activity

I

Ice NEC Y93.29 – *see also* Skiing
- dancing Y93.21
- hockey Y93.22
- skating (figure skating) Y93.21

In-line roller skating (roller blades) Y93.51
Ironing Y93.E4

J

Judo Y93.75
Jumping (off) NEC Y93.39
- BASE jumping (Building, Antenna, Span, Earth) Y93.33
- bungee Y93.34

Jumping jacks Y93.A2
Jumping rope Y93.56

K

Karate Y93.75
Kayaking (in calm and turbulent water) Y93.16
Keyboarding (computer) Y93.C1
- musical instrument J93.J1

Kickball Y93.6A
Knitting Y93.D1

L

Lacrosse Y93.65
Land maintenance NEC Y93.H9 – *see also* Gardening
Landscaping Y93.H2
Laundry Y93.E2
Lifting another person (caregiving) Y93.F2

Note: Use only one activity code. Use these codes only for initial encounter. Do **NOT** use Y93.9 if activity is not documented.

Activity codes – M to R

ACTIVITY codes Y93	
M	**P (continued)**
Machines (exercise)–*see* Exercise(s)	**Polo (water)** Y93.13
Maintenance - *see also* specific activity, such as mopping	**Playing musical instrument**
clothing Y93.E9 – *see also* Laundry	brass instrument Y93.J4
exterior building NEC Y93.H9	drum Y93.J2
household (interior) NEC Y93.E9-	musical keyboard (electronic) Y93.J1
land Y93.H9	percussion instrument NEC Y93.J2
property Y93.H9	piano Y93.J1
Marching (on level or elevated terrain) Y93.01	string instrument Y93.J3
Martial arts Y93.75	wind instrument Y93.J4
Microwave oven Y93.G3	**Property maintenance** - *see also* specific activity such as raking, mopping etc.
Milking an animal Y93.K2	
Mopping (floor) Y93.E5	exterior NEC Y93.H9
Mountain climbing Y93.31	interior NEC Y93.E9
Moving (packing/unpacking while moving to new residence) Y93.E6	**Pruning** (garden and lawn) Y93.H2
	Pull-ups Y93.B2
Muscle-strengthening – *see* Exercise, muscle-Strengthening	**Push-ups** Y93.B2
	R
Musical instrument playing – *see* Playing, musical Instrument	**Racquetball** Y93.73
	Rafting (in calm and turbulent water) Y93.16
Musical keyboard (electronic) playing Y93.J1	**Raking (leaves)** Y93.H1
N	**Rappelling** Y93.32
Nordic skiing Y93.24	**Refereeing a sports activity** Y93.81
O	**Repairing furniture** Y93.D3
Obstacle course Y93.A5	**Repetitive strenuous movements** X50
Other specified activity Y93.89	**Residential relocation** Y93.E6
Oven (microwave) Y93.G3	**Rhythmic gymnastics** Y93.43
Overexertion X50	**Rhythmic movement NEC** Y93.49 - *see also* dancing, gymnastics, etc.
P	
Packing/unpacking in moving to new residence Y93.E6	**Riding horseback** Y93.52
	Rock climbing Y93.31
Parasailing Y93.19	**Roller blades** Y93.51
Pass out game Y93.85	**Rollercoaster riding** Y93.I1
Percussion instrument playing NEC Y93.J2	**Rope jumping** Y93.56
Personal hygiene NEC Y93.E8	**Roller skating (in-line)** (roller blades) Y93.51
bathing and showering Y93.E1	**Rough housing and horseplay** Y93.83
Physical games generally associated with school recess, summer camp and children Y93.6A	**Rowing (in calm and turbulent water)** Y93.16
	Rugby Y93.63
Physical training NEC Y93.A9	**Running** Y93.02
Piano playing Y93.J1	
Pilates Y93.B4	
Platform diving Y93.12	

Note: Do **NOT** use activity codes for poisoning, adverse effects, underdosing, misadventures, sequelae or toxic effects.

Activity codes – S to Y

ACTIVITY codes Y93	
S	**T**
SCUBA diving Y93.15	**Tackle football** Y93.61
Sewing Y93.D2	**Tap dancing** Y93.41
Shearing animal Y93.K3	**Tennis** Y93.73
Shoveling Y93.H1	**Tobogganing** Y93.23
Shoveling Y93.H1	**Track and field events** (other than running) Y93.57
dirt Y93.H1	running Y93.02
snow Y93.H1	**Trampoline** Y93.44
Showering (personal) Y93.E1	**Treadmill** Y93.A1
Sit-ups Y93.B2	**Trimming shrubs** Y93.H2
Skateboarding Y93.51	**Tubing** (in calm and turbulent water) Y93.16
Skating (ice) Y93.21 – *see also* Ice hockey	snow Y93.23
roller Y93.51	**U**
Skiing (alpine) (downhill) Y93.23	**Ultimate frisbee** Y93.74
cross country Y93.24	**Underwater diving** Y93.15
Nordic Y93.24	**Unpacking and moving to new residence** Y93.E6
water Y93.17	**V**
Sledding (snow) Y93.23	**Vacuuming** Y93.E3
Sleeping Y93.84	**Volleyball** (beach) (court) Y93.68
Smoking and grilling food Y93.G2	**W**
Snorkeling Y93.15	**Wake boarding** Y93.17
Snow NEC Y93.29	**Walking** (on level or elevated terrain) Y93.01
boarding Y93.23	an animal Y93.K1
shoveling Y93.H1	**Wall climbing** Y93.31
sledding Y93.23	**Warm up and cool down exercises** Y93.A2
tobogganing Y93.23	**Washing clothes** Y03.E2
tubing Y93.23	**Watching an event** Y93.82
Soccer Y93.66	**Water activity NEC** Y93.19
Softball Y93.64	aerobics Y93.14
Specified activity NEC Y93.89	craft NOS Y93.19
Spectator at an event Y93.82	exercise Y93.14
individual sports NEC Y93.59	parasailing Y93.19
team or group sports NEC Y93.69	polo Y93.13
Springboard diving Y93.12	skiing Y93.17
Squash Y93.73	sliding Y93.18
Stationary bike Y93.A1	survival training and testing Y93.19
stepper machine Y93.A1	wake boarding Y93.17
Stove Y93.G3	**Weeding** (garden and lawn) Y93.H2
Strenuous movements X50	**Wind instrument playing** Y93.J4
String instrument playing V93.J3	**Windsurfing** Y93.18
Surfing Y93.18	**Wrestling** Y93.72
wind Y93.18	**Y**
Swimming Y93.11	**Yoga** Y93.42

Note: Use only one activity code. Use these codes only for initial encounter. Do **NOT** use Y93.9 if activity is not documented.

END OF ACTIVITY CODES

Place of Occurrence A-F

PLACE OF OCCURRENCE Y92

A
Airplane Y92.813
Airport Y92.520
Ambulatory health services establishment NEC Y92.538
Ambulatory surgery center Y92.530
Amusement park Y92.831
Apartment (co-op) —see Place of occurrence, residence, Apartment
Art gallery Y92.250
Assembly hall Y92.29
B
Bank Y92.510
Barn Y92.71
Baseball field Y92.320
Basketball court Y92.310
Beach Y92.832
Bike path Y92.482
Boat Y92.814
Boarding house – see Residence, boarding house
Bowling alley Y92.39
Bridge Y92.89
Building under construction Y92.61
Bus Y92.811
station Y92.521
Business NEC Y92.513
C
Cafe Y92.511
Campsite Y92.833
Campus —see Place of occurrence, school
Canal Y92.89
Car Y92.810
Casino Y92.59
Children's home – see Residence, orphanage
Church Y92.22
Cinema Y92.26
Clubhouse Y92.29
Coal pit Y92.64
College (community) Y92.214
Condominium —see Place of occurrence, residence, apartment

C (continued)
Construction area —see Place of occurrence, industrial and construction area
Convalescent home —see Place of occurrence, residence, nursing home
Court (sports) – see Sports, area, court
Courthouse Y92.240
Cricket ground Y92.328
D
Dancehall Y92.252
Day care center Y92.210
Day nursery Y92.210
Dentist office Y92.531
Derelict house (house in very poor condition) Y92.89
Desert Y92.820
Dock NOS Y92.89
dock Y92.62
dry dock Y92.62
Dockyard Y92.62
Doctor's office Y92.531
Dormitory —see Place of occurrence, residence, school school dormitory
E
Elementary school Y92.211
F
Factory (building) (premises) Y92.63
Farm (land under cultivation) (outbuildings) Y92.79
barn Y92.71
chicken coop Y92.72
farm field – Y92.73 —see also Place of occurrence, residence, farmhouse
hen house Y92.72
specified NEC Y92.79
Field (sports) – see Sports area, field
Football field Y92.321
Forest Y92.821
Freeway Y92.411 – see also Road, Street and Highway

Note: List only one place of occurrence code. Do not use Y92.9 If no place of occurrence is documented.

PLACE OF OCCURRENCE

G

Gallery (art) Y92.250	
Garage (commercial) (used in business) Y92.59	
military base Y92.135	
mobile home Y92.025	
orphanage (children's home) Y92.114	
parking garage Y92.59	
private house (home) Y92.015	
reform school Y92.155	
Gas station Y92.524	
Gasworks Y92.69	
Golf course Y92.39	
Gravel pit Y92.64	
Grocery store Y92.512	
Gymnasium Y92.39	

H

- **Handball court** Y92.318
- **Harbor** Y92.89
- **Harness racing course** Y92.39
- **Healthcare provider's office** Y92.531
- **High school** Y92.213
- **Highway (interstate)** *see* Street and Highway
- **Hill** (wilderness) Y92.828
- **Hockey rink** Y92.330
- **Home** —*see* Place of occurrence, residence
- **Hospice** —*see* Place of occurrence, residence, nursing home
- **Hospital** Y92.239
  - cafeteria Y92.233
  - corridor (hallway) Y92.232
  - operating room Y92.234
  - patient's
    - bathroom Y92.231
    - room Y92.230
  - specified NEC Y92.238
  - unspecified place in hospital Y2.239
- **Hotel** Y92.59
- **House** —*see* Place of occurrence, residence

I

- **Industrial and construction area** (yard) Y92.69

J

- **Jail** – *see* Residence, prison

K

- **Kindergarten** Y92.211

L

- **Lacrosse field** Y92.328
- **Lake** Y92.828
- **Library** Y92.241

M

- **Mall** (shopping) Y92.59
- **Market** Y92.512
- **Marsh** Y92.828
- **Meatpacking facility** Y92.86
- **Middle school** Y92.212
- **Military**
  - base —*see* Place of occurrence, residence, military base
  - training ground Y92.84
- **Mine** Y92.64
- **Mosque** Y92.22
- **Motel** Y92.59
- **Motorway** (interstate) Y92.411
- **Mountain** Y92.828
- **Movie theatre** Y92.26
- **Museum** Y92.251
- **Music hall** Y92.252

N

- **Nuclear power station** Y92.69
- **Nursing home** – *see* Residence, nursing home

O

- **Oil rig** Y92.65
- **Office building** Y92.59
- **Offshore installation** (oil rig) Y92.65
- **Orphanage** —*see* Place of occurrence, residence, orphanage
- **Old people's home** —*see* Place of occurrence, residence, specified NEC
- **Opera house** Y92.253
- **Orchard** Y92.74

Notes: List place of occurrence codes after other External cause codes. **Use these codes only for initial encounter.**

Place of Occurrence P-R

PLACE OF OCCURRENCE

P	R (continued)
Pit Y92.64	**Residence** (home) Y92.009 (continued)
Power station Y92.69	children's home – *see* Orphanage
Park (public) Y92.830	home – *see* House
amusement Y92.831	farmhouse – *see also* Farm Y92.01-
Parking garage Y92.59	bathroom Y92.012
lot Y92.481	bedroom Y92.013
Parkway Y92.412 – *see also* Street, Road, Highway	dining room Y92.011
Pavement Y92.480	driveway Y92.014
Physician's office Y92.531	garage Y92.015
Polo field Y92.328	garden Y92.017
Pond Y92.828	kitchen Y92.010
Post office Y92.242	specified NEC Y92.018
Prairie Y92.828	swimming pool Y92.016
Prison —*see* Place of occurrence, residence, prison	yard Y92.017
Public building – *see also* specific building (library, courthouse, etc.	hospice —*see* Place of occurrence, residence, nursing home
administration building Y92.248	house, single family Y92.019
city hall Y92.243	bathroom Y92.012
hall Y92.29	bedroom Y92.013
other specified NEC Y92.248	dining room Y92.011
R	driveway Y92.014
Race course Y92.39	garage Y92.015
Radio station Y92.59	garden Y92.017
Railway line (bridge) (track) Y92.85	kitchen Y92.010
Ranch (outbuildings) —*see* Place of occurrence, farm	specified NEC Y92.018
Recreation area Y92.838 – *see also* specific area (amusement park, beach, etc.)	swimming pool Y92.016
	yard Y92.017
Reform school- *see* Place of occurrence, residence, reform school	jail – *see* Residence, prison
	military base Y92.139 – *see also* Military training grounds
Religious institution Y92.22	barracks Y92.133
Residence (home) Y92.009	garage Y92.135
apartment (condominium) Y92.039	garden Y92.137
bathroom Y92.031	kitchen Y92.130
bedroom Y92.032	mess hall Y92.131
kitchen Y92.030	specified NEC Y92.138
specified NEC Y92.038	swimming pool Y92.136
boarding house Y92.049	yard Y92.137
bathroom Y92.041	
bedroom Y92.042	
dining room Y92.048	
driveway Y92.043	
garage Y92.044	
garden Y92.046	
kitchen Y92.040	
specified NEC Y92.048	
swimming pool Y92.045	
yard Y92.046	

Notes: List only one place of occurrence code. Do not use Y92.9 if no place of occurrence is documented

PLACE OF OCCURRENCE

Place of Occurrence – Residence (continued)

R (continued)	R (continued)
Residence (home) (continued)	**Residence** (home) (continued)
mobile home Y92.029	reform school Y92.159
bathroom Y92.022	bathroom Y92.152
bedroom Y92.023	bedroom Y92.153
dining room Y92.021	dining room Y92.151
driveway Y92.024	driveway Y92.154
garage Y92.025	garage Y92.155
garden Y92.027	garden Y92.157
kitchen Y92.020	kitchen Y92.150
specified NEC Y92.028	specified NEC Y92.158
swimming pool Y92.026	swimming pool Y92.156
yard Y92.027	yard Y92.157
nursing home Y92.129	residence (home) NEC Y92.198
bathroom Y92.121	bathroom Y92.192
bedroom Y92.122	bedroom Y92.193
dining room Y92.128	dining room Y92.191
driveway Y92.123	driveway Y92.194
garage Y92.124	garage Y92.195
garden Y92.126	garden Y92.197
kitchen Y92.120	kitchen Y92.190
specified NEC Y92.128	specified NEC Y92.198
swimming pool Y92.125	swimming pool Y92.196
yard Y92.126	yard Y92.197
orphanage Y92.119	residence NOS (private) (non-institutional) Y92.009
bathroom Y92.111	bathroom Y92.002
bedroom Y92.112	bedroom Y92.003
dining hall Y92.118	dining room Y92.001
driveway Y92.113	driveway Y92.008
garage Y92.114	garage Y92.008
garden Y92.116	garden Y92.007
kitchen Y92.110	kitchen Y92.000
specified NEC Y92.118	swimming pool Y92.008
swimming pool Y92.115	yard Y92.007
yard Y92.116	school dormitory Y92.169
prison Y92.149 – *see also* Reform school	bathroom Y92.162
bathroom Y92.142	bedroom Y92.163
cell Y92.143	dining room Y92.161
courtyard Y92.147	driveway Y92.168
dining room Y92.141	garage V92.168
kitchen Y92.140	garden V92.168
specified NEC Y92.148	kitchen Y92.160
swimming pool Y92.146	specified NEC Y92.168
	swimming pool Y92.168
	yard Y92.168

Notes: List place of occurrence codes after other External cause codes. **Use these codes only for initial encounter.**

PLACE OF OCCURRENCE

R	
Rest stop (highway) Y92.523	
Restaurant Y92.511	
Riding school Y92.39	
River Y92.828	
Road Y92.410 – see also Street and Highway	
Rodeo ring Y92.39	
Rugby field Y92.328	

S	
Same day surgery center Y92.530	
Sand pit Y92.64	
School (private) (public) (state) Y92.219	
	college Y92.214
	daycare center Y92.210
	elementary school Y92.211
	high school Y92.213
	kindergarten Y92.211
	middle school Y92.212
	other specified school Y92.218
	specified school NEC Y92.218
	trade school Y92.215
	university Y92.214
	unspecified school Y92.219
	vocational school Y92.215
Seashore Y92.832	
Senior citizen center Y92.29	
Shipyard Y92.62	
Shop (commercial) (business) Y92.513	
Shopping mall Y92.59	
Sidewalk Y92.480	
Silo Y92.79	
Skating rink (roller) Y92.331	
	ice Y92.330
Slaughter house Y92.86	
Specified place NEC Y92.89	
Sports area (athletic) – see specific type Y92.39	
	court – see specific type (basketball, tennis, etc.)
	field – see specific type (baseball, soccer)
Store Y92.512	
Stream Y92.828	

S (continued)	
Street and highway Y92.410 – see also Road, Parkway	
	entrance ramp Y92.415
	exit ramp Y92.415
	freeway Y92.411
	highway ramp Y92.415
	interstate highway Y92.411
	local residential or business street Y92.414
	parkway Y92.412
	specified NEC Y92.488
	state road Y92.413
Subway car Y92.816	
Supermarket Y92.512	
Swamp Y92.828	
Swimming pool (public) Y92.34 – see also Residence, specific place, swimming pool	
Synagogue Y92.22	

T	
Television station Y92.59	
Tennis court Y92.312	
Theater (live) Y92.254	
	movie Y92.26
Trade area Y92.59 – see also specific business (bank, garage, hotel, etc.)	
Trade school Y92.215	
Train Y92.815	
	station Y92.522
Truck Y92.812 – see also Accidents, transport	
Tunnel under construction Y92.69	

U	
University Y92.214	
Urgent (health) care center Y92.532	

V	
Vocational school Y92.15	

W	
Warehouse Y92.59	
Water reservoir Y92.89	
Wilderness area Y92.828 - see also specific area (desert, prairie, swamp, etc.)	
Workshop Y92.69	

Y	
Yard, private Y92.096 – see also Residence, place (boarding home, orphanage, etc.)	
Youth center Y92.29	

Z	
Zoo (zoological garden) Y92.834	

Note: List only one place of occurrence code. Do not use Y92.9 If no place of occurrence is documented.

Note: List place of occurrence codes after other External cause codes. **Use these codes only for initial encounter.**

STATUS OF EXTERNAL CAUSE

Status of external cause (role of the patient or patient's activity at the time of the injury) Y99
Hobby not done for income (pay) (salary) Y99.8
Leisure activity (unpaid) Y99.8
Military personnel
military activity (on duty) Y99.1
off-duty activity Y99.8
Recreation or sport not for income (pay) (salary) or while a student Y99.8
Specified NEC Y99.8
Student activity (unpaid) Y99.8
Volunteer activity (unpaid) Y99.2
Work for pay (salary) – civilian
child or other family member performing paid work for family (business) Y99.8
civilian activity done for income or pay Y99.0

Notes: Do **NOT** use status codes for poisoning, adverse effects, underdosing, toxic effects, subsequent visits or sequelae
Use only one status code.

Use for initial encounter only and only if other external cause codes are used.

Do **NOT** use code Y99.9 if no status is documented.

Air and Space Transport Accidents – A-G

CATEGORY – INTENT/CAUSE - ACCIDENTS - Transport
Air and Space Vehicles V95-V97

A	
Aircraft NEC V97.89-	
	machinery in aircraft (injured by) V97.89-
B	
Balloon (nonpowered) V96.00-	
	patient inside/on balloon (injured by)
	collision V96.03-
	crash V96.01-
	explosion V96.05-
	falling from, in or on aircraft V96.00-
	fire V96.04-
	forced landing V96.02-
	specified accident NEC V96.09-
	collision V96.03-
	patient on ground (injured by) balloon
	injury NEC involving balloon V97.39-
	struck by object falling from balloon (includes injury from crash) V97.31-
	while boarding or alighting balloon V97.1-
C	
Commercial aircraft (fixed wing) V95.30-	
	patient inside/on aircraft (injured) (by)
	collision V95.33-
	crash V95.31-
	explosion V95.35-
	falling from, in or on aircraft V95.30-
	fire V95.34-
	forced landing V95.32-
	machinery on aircraft V97.89-
	specified accident NEC V95.30-
	patient on ground (injured by)
	injury NEC with aircraft involvement V97.39-
	rotating propeller V97.32-
	struck by object falling from aircraft (includes injury from crash0 V97.31-
	sucked into aircraft engine V97.33-
	while boarding or alighting aircraft V97.1-

G	
Glider (powered) (includes ultralight, microlight) V95.10-	
	patient inside/on glider (injured by)
	collision V95.13-
	crash V95.11-
	explosion V95.15-
	falling from, in or on aircraft V95.19-
	fire V95.14-
	forced landing V95.12-
	machinery on aircraft V97.89-
	specified accident NEC V95.19-
	machinery on aircraft V97.89-
	patient was on ground (injured by)
	injury NEC involving glider V97.39-
	struck by object falling from glider (includes crash V79.31-
	sucked into glider jet V97.33-
	while boarding or alighting aircraft V97.1-
Glider (nonpowered) V96.20-	
	patient inside/on glider (injured by)
	collision V96.23-
	crash V96.21-
	explosion V96.25-
	falling from, in or on aircraft V96.20-
	fire V96.24-
	forced landing V96.22-
	specified accident NEC V96.29-
	patient on ground (injured) (by)
	injury NEC involving glider V97.39-
	struck by object falling from glider (includes injury from crash) V97.31-
	while boarding or alighting balloon V97.1-

These codes are used for <u>accidental</u> injuries. Do not use if accident is due to military or war operations, legal Intervention, or medical treatment/complication.

Air and Space Transport Accidents – H-U

CATEGORY – INTENT/CAUSE - ACCIDENTS - Transport
Air and Space Vehicles V95-V97

H			P		
Hang glider (nonpowered) V96.19-			**Parachute** V97.29-		
	patient inside/on hang glider (injured by)			patient entangled in object V97.21-	
		collision V96.13-			patient injured on landing V97.22-
		crash V96.11-			patient landed in tree V97.21-
		explosion V96.15-			patient on ground injured by parachute NEC V97.39-
		falling from, in or on aircraft V96.00-			while boarding or alighting balloon V97.1-
		fire V96.14-		**Private aircraft (powered)** (fixed wing) V95.20-	
		forced landing V96.12-			patient inside/on aircraft (injured by)
		specified accident NEC V96.19-			collision V95.23-
	patient on ground (injured) (by) hang glider				crash V95.21-
		injury NEC involving hang glider V97.39-			explosion V95.25-
		struck by object falling from hang glider (includes injury from crash) V97.31-			falling from, in or on aircraft V95.29-
					fire V95.24-
	while boarding or alighting hang glider V97.1-				forced landing V95.22-
Helicopter V95.00-					machinery on aircraft V97.89-
	patient inside/on helicopter (injured by)				specified type NEC V95.29-
	collision V95.03-			patient on ground (injured by)	
	crash V95.01-				injury NEC involving aircraft V97.39-
	explosion V95.05-				rotating propeller V97.32-
	falling from, in or on aircraft V95.09-				struck by object falling from aircraft (includes crash) V79.31-
	fire V95.04-				sucked into aircraft jet V97.33-
	forced landing V95.02-			while boarding or alighting aircraft V97.1-	
	machinery on aircraft V97.89-		S		
	specified accident NEC V95.09-		**Spacecraft**		
	patient was on ground (injured) (by)			patient was inside/on (injured) (by) V95.40-	
		injury NEC involving helicopter (includes crash) V97.39-			collision V95.43-
					crash V95.41-
		rotating propeller V97.32-			explosion V95.45-
		struck by object falling from helicopter V97.31-			falling from, in or on aircraft V95.49-
					fire V95.44-
	while boarding or alighting helicopter V97.1-				forced landing V95.42-
K					specified type NEC V95.49-
Kite (carrying person) (any accident) V96.8-				patient was on ground (injured) (by)	
M					injury NEC involving spacecraft V97.39-
Microlight – see powered aircraft, ultralight					struck by object falling from spacecraft (includes crash) V97.31-
Military aircraft NEC V97.818-					
	civilian injured by V97.811-			while boarding or alighting spacecraft V97.1-	
	collided with civilian aircraft V97.810-		**Specified aircraft NEC** V95.8-		
O			U		
Other specified nonpowered aircraft V96.8-			**Ultralight** – see Glider		
Other specified powered aircraft V95.8-			**Unspecified aircraft accident** V95.9-		

Note: List intent/cause of injury codes before other External Cause codes. Use more than one code if needed to completely explain the circumstances. **Use these codes throughout treatment with applicable 7th character.**

Land Transport Accidents, Nontraffic – Agricultural - Animal-drawn vehicle

CATEGORY – INTENT/CAUSE - ACCIDENTS - Transport
Land – NONTRAFFIC V00-V89

A

Agricultural vehicle (includes tractor, harvester, trailer) trailer) V84.9- (Excludes animal-powered vehicle)	Animal-drawn vehicle (includes horse-drawn carriages, donkey-carts, dogsleds) V80.929-

Agricultural vehicle (includes tractor, harvester, trailer) trailer) V84.9- (Excludes animal-powered vehicle)
- injury (due to) (while)
  - airbag W22.1-
  - boarding or alighting vehicle V84.4-
  - cell phone use Y93.C2
  - vehicle fire X01.0-
  - vehicle stationary or in maintenance W30.81-
- patient was DRIVER V84.5-
- patient was HANGER-ON V84.7-
- patient was OCCUPANT V84.9-
- patient was PASSENGER V84.6-

All-terrain vehicle (includes go cart, golf cart or off-road vehicle) – V86.99 - see also specific vehicle
- injury (due to) (while)
  - airbag W22.1-
  - boarding or alighting V86.45-
  - cell phone use Y93.C2
  - vehicle fire X01.0-
  - vehicle stationary or in maintenance W31-
- patient was DRIVER V86.55-
- patient was HANGER ON V86.75-
- patient was OCCUPANT V86.95-
- patient was PASSENGER V86.65-

Ambulance (any accident) V86.91-
- injury (due to) (while)
  - airbag W22.1-
  - boarding or alighting ambulance V86.41-
  - cell phone use Y93.C2
  - vehicle stationary or in maintenance W31-
  - vehicle fire X01.0-
- patient was DRIVER V86.51-
- patient was HANGER ON V86.71-
- patient was OCCUPANT V86.91-
- patient was PASSENGER V86.61-

Animal-drawn vehicle (includes horse-drawn carriages, donkey-carts, dogsleds) V80.929-
- collided (with)
  - animal V80.12-
    - being ridden V80.711-
  - animal-drawn vehicle (two animal-drawn vehicles collided) V80.721-
  - bus V80.42-
  - car V80.42-
  - fixed or stationary object V80.82-
  - heavy transport vehicle V80.42-
  - hoverboard V80.52-
  - military vehicle V80.910-
  - motorcycle V80.32-
  - other motor vehicle V80.52-
  - other nonmotor vehicle V80.791-
  - pedal cycle V80.22-
  - pedestrian (on foot or using conveyance) V80.12-
  - pick-up truck V80.42-
  - railway vehicle (train) V80.62-
  - Segway V80.52-
  - sport utility vehicle V80.42-
  - streetcar V80.731-
  - three-wheeled motor vehicle V80.32-
  - truck V80.42-
  - van V80.42-
- injury (due to) (while)
  - cell phone use Y93.C2
  - vehicle fire X01.0-
- noncollision accident V80.02-
- other accident V80.928-
- unspecified accident V80.929-

If military vehicle involved, use code for military vehicle, **NOT** type of vehicle. For example, patient was driver of city bus that collided with military truck. Use code for bus driver collided with military vehicle, not collided with truck.

Land Transport Accidents, Nontraffic – Animal-rider - Bulldozer

ACCIDENTS - Transport
Land – NONTRAFFIC V00-V89

A	B
Animal-rider (any animal) V80.919-	**Baby stroller** – (patient in stroller) V00.828-
collided (with)	collided (with)
animal V80.11-	animal V06.09-
being ridden (two riders collided) V80.710-	being ridden V06.09-
animal-drawn vehicle V80.720-	animal-drawn vehicle V06.09-
bus V80.41-	baby stroller (2 strollers collided) V06.09-
car V80.41-	bus V04.09-
fixed or stationary object V80.81-	car V03.09-
heavy transport vehicle V80.41-	fixed or stationary object V00.822-
hoverboard V80.51-	heavy transport vehicle V04.09-
military vehicle V80.910-	hoverboard V09.09-
motorcycle V80.31-	military vehicle V09.01-
other motor vehicle V80.51-	motorcycle V02.09-
other nonmotor vehicle V80.790-	motor vehicle NEC V09.09-
pedal cycle V80.21-	motor vehicle NOS V09.00-
pedestrian (on foot or using conveyance) V80.11-	other nonmotor vehicle V06.09-
pick-up truck V80.41-	pedal cycle V01.09-
railway vehicle (train) V80.61-	pedestrian (on foot or using conveyance) V06.09-
Segway V80.51-	pick-up truck V03.09-
sport utility vehicle V80.41-	railway vehicle (train) V05.09-
streetcar V80.730-	Segway V09.09-
three-wheeled motor vehicle V80.31-	sport utility vehicle V03.09-
truck V80.41-	streetcar V09.09-
van V80.41-	three-wheeled vehicle V02.09-
Injury due to cell phone use Y93.C2	truck V04.09-
noncollision accident (fall from, thrown from)	van V03.09-
patient was riding horse V80.010-	njury due to cell phone use Y93.C2
patient was riding other animal V80.018-	noncollision accident (fall from stroller) V00.821-
other accident V80.918-	other specified accident V00.828-
unspecified accident V80.919-	unspecified accident V00.828-
Armored car — see Accident, nontraffic, truck	**Battery-powered truck** (baggage) – see Accident, transport, nontraffic, Industrial vehicle
	Bicycle – see Accident, transport, nontraffic, pedal cycle
	Bulldozer – see Accident, transport, nontraffic, construction vehicle

These codes are used for <u>accidental</u> injuries. Do not use if injury is due to military or war operations, legal Intervention, or medical treatment/complications.

©2020 Terry Tropin. All Rights Reserved.

Land Transport Accidents, Nontraffic – Bus

ACCIDENTS - Transport
Land – NONTRAFFIC V00-V89

B

Bus (includes motor coach) V79.9-	**Bus** (includes motor coach) (continued) V79.9-
patient was DRIVER	patient was HANGER-ON
collided (with)	collided (with)
animal V70.0-	animal V70.2-
being ridden V76.0-	being ridden V76.2-
animal-drawn vehicle V76.0-	animal-drawn vehicle V76.2-
bus (two buses collided) V74.0-	bus (two buses collided) V74.2-
car V73.0-	car V73.2-
fixed or stationary object V77.0-	fixed or stationary object V77.2-
heavy transport vehicle V74.0-	heavy transport vehicle V74.2-
hoverboard V79.09-	hoverboard V79.29-
military vehicle V79.81-	military vehicle V79.81-
motorcycle V72.0-	motorcycle V72.2-
motor vehicle NEC V79.09-	motor vehicle NEC V79.29-
motor vehicle NOS V79.20-	motor vehicle NOS V79.20-
other nonmotor vehicle V76.0-	other nonmotor vehicle V76.2-
pedal cycle V71.0-	pedal cycle V71.2-
pedestrian (on foot or using conveyance) V70.0-	pedestrian (on foot or sing conveyance) V70.2-
pick-up truck V73.0-	pick-up truck V73.2-
railway vehicle (train) V75.0-	railway vehicle (train) V75.2-
Segway V79.09-	Segway V.79.29-
streetcar V76.0-	sport utility vehicle V73.2-
sport utility vehicle V73.0-	streetcar V76.2-
three wheeled motor vehicle V72.0-	three wheeled motor vehicle V72.2-
truck V74.0-	truck V74.2-
van V73.0-	van V73.2-
injury (due to) (while)	injury (due to) (while)
airbag W22.11-	boarding or alighting bus – see Accident, transport, nontraffic, bus, occupant
boarding or alighting bus – see Accident, transport, nontraffic, bus, occupant	vehicle fire X01.0-
cell phone use Y93.C-	noncollision accident V78.2-
vehicle fire X01.0-	other specified accident V79.88-
noncollision accident V78.0-	unspecified accident V79.3-
other specified accident V79.88-	
unspecified accident V79.3-	

Note: List intent/cause codes before other External Cause codes. Use more than one code if needed to completely explain the circumstances. **Use these codes throughout treatment with applicable 7th character.**

Notes: If military vehicle involved, use code for military vehicle, **NOT** type of vehicle. For example: patient was driver of city bus that hit military truck. Use code for military vehicle, not truck.

ACCIDENTS - Transport
Land – NONTRAFFIC V00-V89

B

Bus (includes motor coach) (continued) V79.9-
- patient was OCCUPANT V79.9-
  - collided (with)
    - animal V70.3-
      - being ridden V76.3-
    - animal-drawn vehicle V76.3-
    - bus (two buses collided) V74.3-
    - car V73.3-
    - fixed or stationary object V77.3-
    - heavy transport vehicle V74.3-
    - hoverboard V79.29-
    - military vehicle V79.81-
    - motorcycle V72.3-
    - motor vehicle NEC V79.29-
    - motor vehicle NOS V79.20-
    - other nonmotor vehicle V76.3-
    - pedal cycle V71.3-
    - pedestrian (on foot or using conveyance) V70.3-
    - pick-up truck V73.3-
    - railway vehicle (train) V75.3-
    - Segway V79.29-
    - sport utility vehicle V73.3-
    - streetcar V76.3-
    - three wheeled motor vehicle V72.3-
    - truck V74.3-
    - van V73.3-
  - injury (due to) (while)
    - airbag W22.1-
    - boarding or alighting bus (collided with) V78.4-
      - animal V70.4-
        - being ridden V76.4-
      - animal-drawn vehicle V76.4-
      - bus V74.4-
      - car V73.4-
      - fixed or stationary object V77.4-
      - heavy transport vehicle V74.4-
      - motorcycle V72.4-
      - other nonmotor vehicle V76.4-
      - pedal cycle V71.4-
      - pedestrian (on foot/conveyance) V70.4-
      - pick-up truck V73.4-
      - railway vehicle (train) V75.4-
      - streetcar V76.4-
      - three wheeled vehicle V72.4-
      - truck V74.3-
      - van V73.4-
    - vehicle fire X01.0-

Bus (includes motor coach) (continued) V79.9-
- patient was OCCUPANT (continued)
  - noncollision accident V78.3-
  - other specified accident V79.88-
  - unspecified accident V79.3-
- patient was PASSENGER
  - collided (with)
    - animal V70.1-
      - being ridden V76.1-
    - animal-drawn vehicle V76.1-
    - bus (two buses collided) V74.1-
    - car V73.1-
    - fixed or stationary object V77.1-
    - heavy transport vehicle V74.1-
    - hoverboard V79.19-
    - military vehicle V79.81-
    - motorcycle V72.1-
    - motor vehicle NEC V79.19-
    - motor vehicle NOS V79.10-
    - other nonmotor vehicle V76.1-
    - pedal cycle V71.1-
    - pedestrian (on foot or using conveyance) V70.1-
    - pick-up truck V73.1-
    - railway vehicle (train) V75.1-
    - Segway V79.19-
    - sport utility vehicle V73.1-
    - streetcar V76.1-
    - three wheeled motor vehicle V72.1-
    - truck V74.1-
    - van V73.1-
  - injury (due to) (while)
    - airbag W22.1-
    - boarding or alighting bus – see Accident, transport, nontraffic, bus, occupant
    - vehicle fire X01.0-
  - noncollision accident V78.1-
  - other specified accident V79.88-
  - unspecified accident V79.3-

These codes are for <u>accidental</u> injuries. Do not use if accident is due to military or war operations, legal intervention, or medical treatment/complication.

©2020 Terry Tropin. All Rights Reserved.

Land Transport Accidents, Nontraffic – Cable car - Car

ACCIDENTS - Transport
Land – NONTRAFFIC V00-V89

C

Cable car (not on rails) V98.0-	**Car** V49.9- (continued)
on rails – see Accident, transport, nontraffic, streetcar	patient was HANGER-ON
Car V49.9-	collided (with)
patient was DRIVER	animal V40.2-
collided (with)	being ridden V46.2-
animal V40.0-	animal-drawn vehicle V46.2-
being ridden V46.0-	bus V44.2-
animal-drawn vehicle V46.0-	car (two cars collided) V43.22-
bus V44.0-	fixed or stationary object V47.2-
car (two cars collided) V43.02-	heavy transport vehicle V44.2-
fixed or stationary object V47.0-	hoverboard V49.29-
heavy transport vehicle V44.0-	military vehicle V49.81-
hoverboard V49.09-	motorcycle V42.2-
military vehicle V49.81-	motor vehicle NEC V49.29-
motorcycle V42.0-	motor vehicle NOS V49.20-
motor vehicle NEC V49.09-	other nonmotor vehicle V46.2-
motor vehicle NOS V49.00-	pedal cycle V41.2-
other nonmotor vehicle V46.0-	pedestrian (on foot/using conveyance) V40.2-
pedal cycle V41.0-	pick-up truck V43.23-
pedestrian (on foot/using conveyance) V4.0-	railway vehicle (train) V45.2-
pick-up truck V43.03-	Segway V49.29-
railway vehicle (train) V45.0-	sport utility vehicle V43.21-
Segway V79.09-	streetcar V46.2-
sport utility vehicle V43.01-	three wheeled motor vehicle V42.2-
streetcar V46.0-	truck V44.2-
three-wheeled motor vehicle V42.0-	van V43.24-
truck V44.0-	injury (due to) (while)
van V43.04-	boarding or alighting car – see Accident, transport, nontraffic, car, occupant
injury (due to) (while)	vehicle fire X01.0-
airbag W22.11-	noncollision accident V48.2-
boarding or alighting car – see Accident, transport, nontraffic, car, occupant	other specified accident V49.88-
cell phone use Y93.C2	unspecified accident V49.3-
vehicle fire X01.0-	
noncollision accident V48.0-	
other specified accident V49.88-	
unspecified accident V49.3-	

Notes: If military vehicle involved, use code for military, **NOT** type of vehicle. For example: patient was car passenger that hit military truck. Use code for military vehicle, not car.

Note: List intent/cause codes before other External Cause codes. Use more than one code if needed to completely explain the circumstances. **Use these codes throughout treatment with applicable 7th character.**

ACCIDENTS - Transport
Land – NONTRAFFIC V00-V89

C (continued)

Car V49.9- (continued)
- patient was OCCUPANT
  - collided (with)
    - animal V40.3-
      - being ridden V46.3-
    - animal-drawn vehicle V46.3-
    - bus V44.3-
    - car (two cars collided) V43.32-
    - fixed or stationary object V47.3-
    - heavy transport vehicle V44.3-
    - hoverboard V49.2-
    - military vehicle V49.81-
    - motorcycle V42.3-
    - motor vehicle NEC V49.29-
    - motor vehicle NOS V49.20-
    - other nonmotor vehicle V46.3-
    - pedal cycle V41.3-
    - pedestrian (on foot or using conveyance) V40.3-
    - pick-up truck V43.33-
    - railway vehicle (train) V45.3-
    - Segway V49.2-
    - sport utility vehicle V43.31-
    - streetcar V46.3-
    - three wheeled motor vehicle V42.3-
    - truck V44.3-
    - van V43.34-
  - injury (due to) (while)
    - airbag W22.10-
    - boarding or alighting car (collided with) V48.4-
      - animal V40.4-
        - being ridden V46.4-
      - animal-drawn vehicle V46.4-
      - bus V44.4-
      - car (two cars collided) V43.42-
      - fixed or stationary object V47.4-
      - heavy transport vehicle V44.4-
      - motorcycle V42.4-
      - other nonmotor vehicle V46.4-
      - pedal cycle V41.4-
      - pedestrian (on foot/using conveyance) V40.4-
      - pick-up truck V43.42-
      - railway vehicle (train) V45.4-
      - sport utility vehicle V43.41-
      - streetcar V46.4-
      - three-wheeled vehicle V42.4-
      - truck V44.4-
      - van V43.44-
    - vehicle fire X01.0-

Car V49.9- (continued)
- patient was OCCUPANT (continued)
  - noncollision accident V48.3-
    - while boarding or alighting car V48.4-
  - other specified accident V49.88-
  - unspecified accident V49.3-
- patient was PASSENGER
  - collided (with)
    - animal V40.1-
      - being ridden V46.1-
    - animal-drawn vehicle V46.1-
    - bus V44.1-
    - car (two cars collided) V43.12-
    - fixed or stationary object V47.1-
    - heavy transport vehicle V44.1-
    - hoverboard V49.19-
    - military vehicle V49.81-
    - motorcycle V42.1-
    - motor vehicle NEC V49.19-
    - motor vehicle NOS V49.10-
    - other nonmotor vehicle V46.1-
    - pedal cycle V41.1-
    - pedestrian (on foot or using conveyance) V40.1-
    - pick-up truck V43.13-
    - railway vehicle (train) V45.1-
    - Segway V49.19-
    - sport utility vehicle V43.11-
    - streetcar V46.1-
    - three wheeled motor vehicle V42.1-
    - truck V44.1-
    - van V43.14-
  - injury (due to) (while)
    - airbag W22.12-
    - boarding or alighting car – see Accident, transport, nontraffic, car, occupant
    - cell phone use Y93.C2
    - vehicle fire X01.0-
  - noncollision accident V48.1-
  - other specified accident V49.88-
  - unspecified accident V49.3-

These codes are used for <u>accidental</u> injuries. Do not use if injury is due to military or war operations, legal intervention, Or medical treatment/complication.

©2020 Terry Tropin. All Rights Reserved.

Land Transport Accidents, Nontraffic – Coal car – Electric Scooter

ACCIDENTS - Transport
Land – NONTRAFFIC V00-V89

C (continued)		E	
Coal car —see Accident, transport, nontraffic, industrial vehicle		**Earth-leveler** - see Accident, transport, nontraffic, construction vehicle	
Construction vehicle (includes bulldozer, digger, dump truck, earth leveler, mechanical shovel)		**Electric scooter (standing) – see also Hoverboard**	
	injury (due to) (while)		collided (with)
	airbag W22.1-		animal (being ridden) V06.031
	boarding or alighting vehicle V85.4-		animal drawn vehicle V06.031
	cell phone use Y93.C2		bus V04.031
	vehicle fire X01.0-		car V03.031
	vehicle stationary or in maintenance W31-		electric scooter (two scooters collide) V06.031
	patient was DRIVER V85.5-		fixed or stationary object V00.842
	patient was HANGER-ON V85.7-		heavy transport vehicle V04.031
	patient was OCCUPANT V85.9-		motorcycle V02.031
	patient was PASSENGER V85.6-		other motor vehicle V06.031
D			other nonmotor vehicle V06.031
Digger – see Accident, transport, nontraffic, construction vehicle			pedal cycle V01.031
Dirt bike (includes motor/cross bike) – see also Accident, transport, nontraffic, all-terrain vehicle			pedestrian (on foot /using conveyance) V06.031
	injury (due to) (while)		railway vehicle (train) V05.031
	boarding or alighting V86.46-		sport utility vehicle V03.031
	cell phone use Y93.C2		streetcar (nonpowered) V06.031
	vehicle fire X01.0-		three-wheeled vehicle V02.031
	vehicle stationary or in maintenance W31-		truck V04.09-
	patient was DRIVER V86.56-		van V03.031
	patient was HANGER ON V86.76-		fell (from) off) V00.841	
	patient was OCCUPANT V86.96-		Injury, due to cell phone use Y93.C2	
	patient was PASSENGER V86.66-			
Dump truck – see Accident, transport, nontraffic, construction vehicle			
Dune buggy			
	injury (due to) (while)		
	boarding or alighting dune buggy V86.43-		
	cell phone use Y93.C2		
	vehicle fire X01.0-		
	patient was DRIVER V86.53-		
	patient was HANGER ON V86.73-		
	patient was OCCUPANT V86.93-		
	patient was PASSENGER V86.V86.63-		

List intent/cause codes before other External Cause codes. Use more than one code if needed to completely explain the circumstances. **Use these codes throughout treatment with applicable 7th character.**

©2020 Terry Tropin. All Rights Reserved.

ACCIDENTS - Transport
Land – NONTRAFFIC V00-V89

F
Farm machinery -see Accident, transport, nontraffic, agricultural vehicle
Fire engine (truck) V86.91-
injury (due to) (while)
airbag W22.1-
boarding or alighting fire engine V86.41-
cell phone use Y93.C2
vehicle fire X01.0-
patient was DRIVER V86.51-
patient was HANGER ON V86.71-
patient was OCCUPANT V86.91-
patient was PASSENGER V86.61-
Forklift – see Accident, transport, nontraffic, industrial vehicle
G
Go cart —see Accident, transport, nontraffic, all-terrain vehicle
Golf cart —see Accident, transport, nontraffic, all-terrain vehicle
H
Harvester - see Accident, transport, nontraffic, agricultural vehicle
Heavy transport vehicle —see Accident, transport, nontraffic, truck or bus
Heelies V00.158-
collided (with)
fixed or stationary object V00.152-
other object or vehicle V00.158-
pedestrian (on foot or using conveyance) V00.158-
fell (from) (off) V00.151-
Injury due to cell phone use Y93.C2
noncollision accident V00.158-

H (continued)
Hoverboard V00.848
collided (with)
animal (being ridden) V06.038
animal drawn vehicle V06.038
bus V04.038
car V03.038
fixed or stationary object V00.842
heavy transport vehicle V04.038
hoverboard (two hoverboards collide) V06.038
motorcycle V02.038
other motor vehicle V06.038
other nonmotor vehicle V06.038
pedal cycle V01.038
pedestrian (on foot or using conveyance) V06.038
pick-up truck V03.038
railway vehicle (train) V05.038
sport utility vehicle V03.038
streetcar (nonpowered) V06.038
three-wheeled vehicle V02.038
truck V04.09-
van V03.038
fell (from) (0ff) V00.848
Injury due to cell phone use Y93.C2

If military vehicle involved, use codes for military vehicle, **NOT** type of vehicle. For example, patient was driver of heavy transport vehicle that collided with military truck. Use code for heavy transport vehicle collided with military vehicle, not truck.

Land Transport Accidents, Nontraffic – Ice skates – Motor/Cross

ACCIDENTS - Transport
Land – NONTRAFFIC V00-V89

I	M
Ice skates V00.218-	**Mechanical shovel** – see transport, nontraffic, construction vehicle
collided (with)	
animal (being ridden) V06.09-	**Military vehicle** V86.94-
bus V04.09-	injury (due to) (while)
car V03.09-	airbag W22.1-
fixed or stationary object V00.212-	boarding or alighting vehicle V86.44-
heavy transport vehicle V04.09-	cell phone use Y93.C2
hoverboard V09.00-	vehicle fire X01.0-
ice skates (two ice skaters collided) V00.218-	patient was DRIVER V86.54-
motorcycle V02.09-	patient was HANGER ON V86.74-
other motor vehicle V09.00-	patient was OCCUPANT V86.94-
other nonmotor vehicle V06.09-	patient was PASSENGER V86.64-
pedal cycle V01.09-	**Mine tram** —see Accident, transport, nontraffic, industrial vehicle
pedestrian (on foot or using conveyance) V06.09-	**Mini-bus**–see Accident, transport, nontraffic, pick-up truck or van
pick-up truck V03.09-	**Mini-van** - see Accident, transport, traffic, pick-up truck or van
railway vehicle (train) V05.09-	**Mobility scooter** (motorized) (driver, passenger, or occupant) V00.838-
Segway V09.00-	collided (with)
sport utility vehicle V03.09-	bus V04.09-
streetcar (nonpowered) V06.09-	car V03.09-
three-wheeled vehicle V02.09-	fixed or stationary object V00.832-
truck V04.09-	heavy transport vehicle V04.09-
van V03.09-	hoverboard V09.09-
fell (from) (off) V00.211-	mobility scooter (two scooters collided) V00.838-
Industrial vehicle (includes battery-powered truck, coal car, forklift, logging car, mine tram) V83.9-	motorcycle V02.09-
injury (due to) (while)	other motor vehicle V09.09-
airbag W22.1-	other nonmotor vehicle V06.09-
boarding or alighting vehicle V83.4-	pedal cycle V01.09-
cell phone use Y93.C2	pedestrian (on foot or using conveyance) V06.09-
vehicle fire X01.0-	pick-up truck V03.09-
vehicle stationary or in maintenance W31.83-	railway vehicle (train) V05.09-
patient was DRIVER V83.5-	Segway V09.09-
patient was HANGER-ON V83.7-	sport utility vehicle V03.09-
patient was OCCUPANT V83.9-	streetcar (nonpowered) V06.09-
patient was PASSENGER V83.6-	three-wheeled vehicle V02.09-
L	truck V04.09-
Logging car —see Accident, transport, nontraffic, industrial vehicle	van V03.09-
	injury (due to)
	airbag W22.1-
	cell phone use Y93.C2
	fall (from) (out) V00.831-
	vehicle fire X01.0-
	other mobility scooter accident V00.838-
	Moped –see Accident, transport, nontraffic, motorcycle
	Motor coach —see Accident, transport, nontraffic, bus
	Motor/cross bike – see Dirt bike

List intent/cause codes before other External Cause codes. Use more than one code if needed to completely explain the circumstances. **Use these codes throughout treatment with applicable 7th character.**

©2020 Terry Tropin. All Rights Reserved.

page 74

ACCIDENTS - Transport
Land – NONTRAFFIC V00-V89

M (continued)

Motorcycle (includes motorized scooter, moped) V29.3-
- patient was DRIVER
  - collided (with)
    - animal V20.0-
      - being ridden V26.0-
    - animal-drawn vehicle V26.0-
    - bus V24.0-
    - car V23.0-
    - fixed or stationary object V27.0-
    - heavy transport V24.0-
    - hoverboard V29.0-
    - military vehicle V29.81-
    - motorcycle (two motorcycles collided) V22.0-
    - other motor vehicle V29.0-
    - other nonmotor vehicle V26.0-
    - pedal vehicle V21.0-
    - pedestrian (on foot or using conveyance) V20.0-
    - pick-up truck V23.0-
    - railway vehicle (train) V25.0-
    - Segway V29.0-
    - sport utility vehicle V23.0-
    - streetcar V26.0-
    - three wheeled motor vehicle V22.0-
    - truck V24.0-
    - van V23.0-
  - injury (due to) (while)
    - boarding or alighting – see Accident, transport, nontraffic, motorcycle, occupant
    - cell phone use Y93.C2
    - vehicle fire X01.0-
  - noncollision accident V28.0-
  - other specified accident V29.88-
  - unspecified accident V29.3-
- patient was OCCUPANT
  - collided (with)
    - animal V20.2-
      - being ridden V26.2-
    - animal-drawn vehicle V26.2-
    - bus V24.2-
    - car V23.2-
    - fixed or stationary object V27.2-
    - heavy transport vehicle V24.2-
    - hoverboard V29.2-
    - military vehicle V29.81-
    - motorcycle (2 motorcycles collided) V22.2-
    - military vehicle V29.81-

M (continued)

Motorcycle (includes motorized scooter, moped) (cont) V29.3-
- patient was OCCUPANT (continued)
  - collided (with) (continued)
    - other motor vehicle V29.2-
    - other nonmotor vehicle V26.2-
    - pedal cycle V21.2-
    - pedestrian (on foot or using conveyance) V20.2
    - pick-up truck V23.2-
    - railway vehicle (train) V25.2-
    - sport utility vehicle V23.2-
    - streetcar V26.2-
    - three wheeled motor vehicle V22.2-
    - truck V24.2
    - van V23.2-
  - injury (due to) (while)
    - boarding or alighting cycle (collided with)
      - animal V20.3-
        - being ridden V26.3-
      - animal-drawn vehicle V26.3-
      - bus V24.3-
      - car V23.3-
      - fixed or stationary object V27.3-
      - heavy transport vehicle V24.3-
      - hoverboard V29.2-
      - military vehicle V29.81-
      - motorcycle (two motorcycles involved) V22.3-
      - other motor vehicle V29.2-
      - other nonmotor vehicle V26.3-
      - pedal cycle V21.3-
      - pedestrian (on foot/using conveyance) V20.3-
      - pick-up truck V23.3-
      - railway vehicle (train) V25.3-
      - Segway V29.2-
      - sport utility vehicle V23.3-
      - streetcar V26.3-
      - three-wheeled vehicle V22.3-
      - truck V24.3-
      - van V23.3-
    - vehicle fire X01.0-
  - noncollision accident V28.2-
    - while boarding or alighting V28.3-
    - other specified accident V29.88-
    - unspecified accident V29.3-

These codes are used <u>for accidental</u> injuries. Do not use if injury is due to military or war operations, legal intervention or medical treatment/complications.

Land Transport Accidents, Nontraffic – Motorcycle – Pedal Cycle

ACCIDENTS - Transport
Land – NONTRAFFIC V00-V89

M (continued)		
Motorcycle (includes motorized scooter, moped) (cont.) V29.3		
	patient was PASSENGER	
		collided (with)
		animal V20.1-
		animal-drawn vehicle V26.1-
		bus V24.1-
		car V23.1-
		fixed or stationary object V27.1-
		heavy transport vehicle V24.1-
		hoverboard V29.19-
		military vehicle V29.81-
		motorcycle (2 motorcycles collided) V22.1-
		motor vehicle NEC V29.19-
		motor vehicle NOS V29.10-
		other nonmotor vehicle V26.1-
		pedal vehicle V21.1-
		pedestrian (on foot or using conveyance) V20.1-
		pick-up truck V23.1-
		railway vehicle (train) V25.1-
		Segway V29.19-
		sport utility vehicle V23.1-
		streetcar V26.1-
		three wheeled motor vehicle V22.1-
		truck V24.1-
		van V23.1-
	injury (due to) (while)	
		boarding or alighting motorcycle – see Accident, Transport, nontraffic, motorcycle, Occupant
		vehicle fire X01.0-
	noncollision accident V28.1-	
		entanglement in wheel V19.88-
		explosion of motorcycle tire W37.8-
	other specified accident V29.88-	
	unspecified accident V29.3-	
Motor vehicle NOS V89.0-		

N	
Nonmotor vehicle NOS V89.1-	
O	
Off road vehicle – see All-terrain vehicle or Motor/cross bike	
P	
Pedal cycle (includes tricycle, bicycle, rickshaw) V19.3-	
	patient was DRIVER
		collided (with)
		animal V10.0-
		animal-drawn vehicle V16.0-
		bus V14.0-
		car V13.0-
		fixed or stationary object V17.0-
		heavy transport vehicle V14.0-
		hoverboard V19.09-
		military vehicle V19.81-
		motor cycle V12.0-
		motor vehicle NEC V19.09-
		motor vehicle NOS V19.00-
		other nonmotor vehicle V16.0-
		pedal cycle (2 pedal cycles collided) V11.0-
		pick-up truck V13.0-
		railway vehicle (train) V15.0-
		Segway V19.09-
		sport utility vehicle V13.0-
		streetcar V16.0-
		three wheeled motor vehicle V12.0-
		truck V14.0-
		van V13.0-
	injury (while)
		boarding or alighting pedal cycle – see Accident, transport, pedal cycle, Occupant
		cell phone use Y93.C2
	noncollision accident V18.0-
		entanglement in wheel V19.88-
		explosion of bicycle tire W37.0-
	other specified accident V19.88-
	unspecified accident V19.3-

Note: List intent/cause codes before other External Cause codes. Use more than one code if needed to completely explain the circumstances. **Use these codes throughout treatment with applicable 7th character.**

Note: If military vehicle involved, use code for military, not type of vehicle. For example, patient on pedal cycle was hit by military motorcycle. Use code for military vehicle, not motorcycle.

Land Transport Accidents, Nontraffic – Pedal Cycle

ACCIDENTS - Transport
Land – NONTRAFFIC V00-V89

P (continued)
Pedal cycle (includes tricycle, bicycle, rickshaw) (cont.) V19.3-
patient was OCCUPANT
collided (with)
animal V10.2-
animal-drawn vehicle V16.2-
bus V14.2-
car V13.2-
fixed or stationary object V17.2-
heavy transport vehicle V14.2-
hoverboard V19.2-
military vehicle V19.81-
motor cycle V12.2-
other motor vehicle V19.2-
other nonmotor vehicle V16.2-
pedal cycle (2 pedal cycles collided) V11.2-
pedestrian (on foot/using conveyance) V10.2-
pick-up truck V13.2-
railway vehicle (train) V15.2-
Segway V19.2-
sport utility vehicle V13.2-
streetcar V16.2-
three wheeled motor vehicle V12.2-
truck V14.2-
van V13.2-
injury (while)
boarding or alighting pedal cycle (collided with)
animal V10.3-
animal-drawn vehicle V16.3-
bus V14.3-
car V13.3-
fixed or stationary object V17.3-
heavy transport vehicle V14.3-
motorcycle V12.3-
other nonmotor vehicle V16.3-
pedal cycle (2 cycles collided) V11.3-
pedestrian (on foot/using conveyance) V10.3-
pick-up truck V13.3-
railway vehicle (train) V15.3-
sport utility vehicle V13.3-
streetcar V16.3-
three-wheeled vehicle V12.3-
truck V14.3-
van V13.3-

P (continued)
Pedal cycle (includes tricycle, bicycle, rickshaw) (cont.) V19.3-
patient was OCCUPANT (continued)
noncollision accident V18.2-
entanglement in wheel V19.88-
explosion of bicycle tire W37.0-
while boarding or alighting cycle V18.3-
other specified accident V19.88-
unspecified accident V19.3-
patient was PASSENGER
collided (with)
animal V10.1-
animal-drawn vehicle V16.1-
bus V14.1-
car V13.1-
fixed or stationary object V17.1-
heavy transport vehicle V14.1-
hoverboard V19.19-
military vehicle V19.81-
motorcycle V12.1-
other motor vehicle V19.19-
other nonmotor vehicle V16.10-
pedal cycle (two cycles collided) V11.1-
pedestrian (on foot/using conveyance) V10.1-
pick-up truck V13.1-
railway vehicle (train) V15.1-
Segway V19.19-
sport utility vehicle V13.1-
streetcar V16.1-
three wheeled motor vehicle V12.1-
truck V14.1
van V13.1-
injury (while)
boarding or alighting pedal cycle – see Accident transport, nontraffic, pedal cycle, Occupant
noncollision V18.1-
entanglement in wheel V19.88-
explosion of bicycle tire W37.0-
while boarding or alighting cycle V18.3-
other specified accident V19.88-
unspecified accident V19.3-

These codes are used for <u>accidental</u> injuries. Do not use if injury is due to military or war operations, legal interventions or medical treatment/complications.

Land Transport Accidents, Nontraffic – Pedestrian-Pedestrian conveyance

ACCIDENTS - Transport
Land – NONTRAFFIC V00-V89

P (continued)	P (continued)
Pedestrian (on foot) – see also Fall, Slipping V09.1-	**Pedestrian conveyance** – see also specific conveyance (roller skates, baby stroller, hoverboard, etc.) V09.9-
collided (with)	collided with other land transport vehicle – see V01-V09 with 5th character 9
animal – see Contact, with, animal, struck by	
being ridden V06.00-	flat-bottomed pedestrian conveyance NEC – see also snowboard or skis (snow) V00.388-
animal-drawn vehicle V06.00-	
bus V04.00-	collided (with)
car V03.00-	fixed or stationary object V00.382-
fixed or stationary object –see Fall, Striking against, etc.	other vehicle or object V00.388-
heavy transport vehicle V04.00-	other flat-bottomed conveyances V00.388-
hoverboard V00.038	fell (from) (on) (off) flat-bottomed conveyance V00.381-
military vehicle V09.01-	gliding-type pedestrian conveyance NEC – see also ice skates or sled V00.288-
motorcycle V02.00-	
motor vehicle NEC V09.09-	collided (with)
motor vehicle NOS V09.00-	fixed or stationary object V00.282-
other nonmotor vehicle V06.00-	other vehicle or object V00.388-
pedal cycle V01.00-	other gliding-type conveyance V00.388-
pedestrian (two pedestrians collided) W51-	fell (from) (on) (off) gliding conveyance V00.281-
with fall W03-	rolling-type pedestrian conveyance NEC – see also roller skates, skateboard, scooter V00.188
due to ice or snow W00.0-	
pedestrian conveyance NEC V00.09-	collided (with)
pick-up truck V03.00-	fixed or stationary object V00.182-
railway vehicle (train) V05.00-	other vehicle or object V00.388-
roller skater V00.01-	other gliding-type conveyance V00.388-
Segway V00.038	fell (from) (on) (off) rolling conveyance V00.181-
skateboarder V00.02-	unspecified pedestrian conveyance V00.898-
sport utility vehicle V03.00-	collided (with)
streetcar (nonpowered) V06.00-	fixed or stationary object V00.892-
standing	other vehicle or object V00.388-
electric scooter V00.031	other gliding-type conveyance V00.388-
micro-mobility pedestrian conveyance NEC V00.038-	fell (from) (on) (off) conveyance V00.891-
three-wheeled motor vehicle V02.00-	injury due to cell phone use Y93.C2
truck V04.00-	
van V03.00-	
injury due to cell phone use Y93.C2	
noncollision accident – see Fall, Slipping, etc.	
unspecified pedestrian accident V09.1-	

List intent/cause codes before other External Cause codes. Use more than one code if needed to completely explain the circumstances. Use these codes throughout treatment with applicable 7th character.

If military vehicle involved, use code for military, not type of vehicle. For example, pedestrian was hit by military motorcycle. Use code for pedestrian hit by military vehicle, not motorcycle.

Land Transport Accidents, Nontraffic – Pick-up Truck or Van

ACCIDENTS - Transport
Land – NONTRAFFIC V00-V89

P (continued)
Pick-up truck or van – V59.3- see also Truck (includes minibus, minivan, sport utility vehicle)
patient was DRIVER
collided (with)
animal V50.0-
being ridden V56.0-
animal-drawn vehicle V56.0-
bus V54.0-
car V53.0-
fixed or stationary object V57.0-
heavy transport vehicle V54.0-
hoverboard V59.09-
military vehicle V59.81-
motorcycle V52.0-
motor vehicle NEC V59.09-
motor vehicle NOS V59.00-
other nonmotor vehicle V56.0-
pedal cycle V51.0-
pedestrian (on foot or using conveyance) V50.0-
pick-up truck (2 pick-up trucks or pick-up truck and van collided) V53.0-
railway vehicle (train) V55.0-
Segway V59.09-
sport utility vehicle V53.0-
streetcar V56.0-
three wheeled motor vehicle V52.0-
truck V54.0-
van (2 vans or pick-up truck and van collided) V53.0-
injury (due to) (while)
airbag W22.11-
boarding or alighting pick-up truck or van - *see* Accident, transport, pick-up truck or van, occupant
cell phone use Y93.C2
vehicle fire X01.0-
noncollision V58.0-
other specified accident V59.88-
unspecified accident V59.3-

Note: List intent/cause codes before other External Cause codes. Use more than one code if needed to completely explain the circumstances. **Use these codes throughout treatment with applicable 7th character.**

P (continued)
Pick-up truck or van – V59.3- see *also* Truck. (Includes minibus, minivan, sport utility vehicle (continued)
patient was HANGER-ON
collided (with)
animal V50.2-
being ridden V56.2-
animal-drawn vehicle V56.2-
bus V54.2-
car V53.2-
fixed or stationary object V57.2-
heavy transport vehicle V54.2-
hoverboard V59.29-
military vehicle V59.81-
motorcycle V52.2-
motor vehicle NEC V59.29-
motor vehicle NOS V59.20-
other nonmotor vehicle V56.2-
pedal cycle V51.2-
pedestrian (on foot or using conveyance) V50.2-
pick-up truck (2 pick-up trucks or pick-up truck and van collided) V53.2-
railway vehicle (train) V55.2-
Segway V59.29-
sport utility vehicle V53.2-
streetcar V56.2-
three wheeled motor vehicle V52.2-
truck V54.2-
van (2 vans or van and pick-up truck collided) V53.2-
injury (due to) (while)
boarding or alighting pick-up truck or van - *see* Accident, transport, pick-up truck or van, occupant
vehicle fire X01.0-
noncollision accident V58.2-
other specified accident V59.88-
unspecified accident V59.3-

Note: These codes are for <u>accidental</u> injuries. Do not use if injury due to military or war operations, legal intervention, complication, or misadventure.

ACCIDENTS - Transport
Land – NONTRAFFIC V00-V89

P (continued)	P (continued)
Pick-up truck or van – V59.3- - see also truck. (Includes minibus, minivan, sport utility vehicle) (continued)	**Pick-up truck or van** – V59.3- see also truck. (Includes minibus, minivan, sport utility vehicle) (continued)

Pick-up truck or van – V59.3- - see also truck. (Includes minibus, minivan, sport utility vehicle) (continued)
- patient was OCCUPANT
  - collided (with)
    - animal V50.3-
      - being ridden V56.3-
    - animal-drawn vehicle V56.3-
    - bus V54.3-
    - car V53.3-
    - fixed or stationary object V57.3-
    - heavy transport vehicle V54.3-
    - hoverboard V59.2-
    - military vehicle V59.81-
    - motorcycle V52.3-
    - other motor vehicle V59.2-
    - other nonmotor vehicle V56.3-
    - pedal cycle V51.3-
    - pedestrian (on foot/using conveyance) V50.3-
    - pick-up truck (two pick-up trucks or pick-up truck and van collided) V53.3-
    - railway vehicle (train) V55.3-
    - Segway V59.2-
    - sport utility vehicle V53.3-
    - streetcar V56.3-
    - three wheeled motor vehicle V52.3-
    - truck V54.3-
    - van (two vans or van and pick-up truck collided) collided) V53.3-
  - injury (due to) (while)
    - airbag W22.19-
    - boarding or alighting pick-up truck/van (collided with)
      - animal V50.4-
        - being ridden V56.4-
      - animal-drawn vehicle V56.4-
      - bus V54.4-
      - car V53.4-
      - fixed or stationary object V57.4-
      - heavy transport vehicle V54.4-
      - motorcycle V52.4-
      - other nonmotor vehicle V56.4-
      - pedal cycle V51.4-
      - pedestrian (on foot/using conveyance) V50.4-
      - pick-up truck V53.4-
      - railway vehicle (train) V55.4-
      - sport utility vehicle V53.4-
      - streetcar V56.4-

Pick-up truck or van – V59.3- see also truck. (Includes minibus, minivan, sport utility vehicle) (continued)
- patient was OCCUPANT (continued)
  - injury (due to) (while)
    - boarding or alighting (collided with) (cont.)
      - three-wheeled vehicle V52.4-
      - truck V54.4-
      - van V53.4-
      - vehicle fire X01.0-
    - noncollision accident V58.3-
      - while boarding or alighting V58.4-
    - other specified accident V59.69-
    - unspecified accident V59.60-
- patient was PASSENGER
  - collided (with)
    - animal V50.1-
      - being ridden V56.1-
    - animal-drawn vehicle V56.1-
    - bus V54.1-
    - car V53.1-
    - fixed or stationary object V57.1-
    - heavy transport vehicle V54.1-
    - hoverboard V59.1-
    - military vehicle V59.81-
    - motorcycle V52.1-
    - other motor vehicle V59.1-
    - other nonmotor vehicle V56.1-
    - pedal cycle V51.1-
    - pedestrian (on foot/using conveyance) V50.1-
    - pick-up truck (2 pick-up trucks/pick-up truck and van) V53.1-
    - railway vehicle (train) V55.1-
    - Segway V59.1-
    - sport utility vehicle V53.1-
    - streetcar V56.1-
    - three wheeled motor vehicle V52.1-
    - truck V54.1-
    - van (two vans/van & pick-up truck collided) V53.1-
  - injury (due to) (while)
    - airbag W22.12-
    - boarding or alighting – see Accident, transport, Non-traffic, pick-up truck or van, occupant
    - vehicle fire X01.0-
  - noncollision accident V58.1-
  - other specified accident V59.29-
  - unspecified accident V59.20-

Land Transport Accidents, Nontraffic – Railway vehicle – Roller Skates (in-line)

ACCIDENTS - Transport
Land – NONTRAFFIC V00-V89

R	R (continued)
Railway vehicle (train) (includes subway an elevated train) V81.9- see *also* Streetcar	**Roller skates (in-line)** (roller blades) V00.118- – see also Roller skates (other than inline)
patient was OCCUPANT (may be engineer, conductor, other crew, passenger or hanger-on)	patient was OCCUPANT
collided (with)	collided (with)
animal V81.3-	animal being ridden V06.01-
being ridden V81.3-	animal-drawn vehicle V06.01-
fixed or stationary object V81.3-	bus V04.01-
military vehicle V81.83-	car V03.01-
motor vehicle V81.0-	fixed or stationary object V00.112-
nonmotor vehicle V81.3-	heavy transport vehicle V04.01-
other object V81.3-	military vehicle V09.01-
rolling stock V81.2-	motorcycle V02.01-
railway vehicle (train) V81.2-	other land transport vehicle – see V01-V09 with 5th character 9
injury (due to (while))	other nonmotor vehicle V06.01-
boarding or alighting V81.4-	other object/person V00.118-
derailment of train	pedal cycle V01.01-
without collision V81.7-	pedestrian (on foot or using conveyance) V00.118-
fall after derailment V81.3-	pick-up truck V03.01-
explosion V81.81-	railway vehicle (train) V05.01-
fall V81.5-	roller skates (two skaters collide) V06.118-
after derailment V81.3-	sport utility vehicle V03.01-
during derailment V81.7-	streetcar (nonpowered) V06.01-
fall <u>in</u> train V81.5-	three wheeled vehicle V02.01-
fall <u>from</u> train V81.6-	truck V04.01-
object falling onto train (earth, rocks, stones, etc.) V81.82-	van V03.01-
vehicle fire V81.81-	fall (from) (off) V00.111-
other specified accident V81.89-	noncollision accident V00.118-
unspecified accident V81.9-	other accident V00.118-
Rickshaw – see Accident, transport, nontraffic, pedal cycle	unspecified accident V00.118-
Roller blades – see Roller skates (in-line)	

List intent/cause codes before other External Cause codes. Use more than one code if needed to completely explain the circumstances. **Use these codes throughout treatment with applicable 7th character.**

If military vehicle involved, use code for military, not type of vehicle. For example, roller skater hit by military truck. Use code for roller skater hit by military vehicle, not truck.

Land Transport Accidents, Nontraffic – Roller skates (other than in-line) – Scooter

ACCIDENTS - Transport
Land – NONTRAFFIC V00-V89

R (continued)	S (continued)
Roller skates (other than in-line) V00.128 – see also Roller skates (in-line)	**Scooter (nonmotorized)** V00.148- (driver, occupant, or passenger) If motorized, see Motorcycle, Mobility scooter, Electric scooter or Hoverboard
collided (with)	collided (with)
animal V06.01-	animal being ridden V06.09-
being ridden V06.01-	animal-drawn vehicle V06.09-
animal-drawn vehicle V06.01-	bus V04.09-
bus V04.01-	car V03.09-
car V03.01-	fixed or stationary object V00.142-
fixed or stationary object V00.122-	heavy transport vehicle V04.09-
heavy transport vehicle V04.01-	military vehicle V09.01-
military vehicle V09.01-	motorcycle V02.09-
motorcycle V02.01-	other land transport vehicle – *see* V01-V09 with 5th character 9
other land transport vehicle – *see* V01-V09 with 5th character 9	other nonmotor vehicle V06.09-
other nonmotor vehicle V06.01-	pedal cycle V01.09-
pedal cycle V01.01-	pedestrian (on foot or using conveyance) V06.09-
pedestrian (on foot or using conveyance) V00.128-	pick-up truck V03.09-
pick truck V03.01-	railway vehicle (train) V05.09-
railway vehicle (train) V05.01-	scooter (nonmotorized) (two scooters collided) V06.09-
roller skates (two skaters collide) V00.128-	sport utility vehicle V03.09-
sport utility vehicle V03.01-	streetcar (nonpowered) V06.09-
streetcar (nonpowered) V06.01-	three-wheeled vehicle V02.09-
three-wheeled vehicle V02.01-	truck V04.09-
truck V04.01-	van V03.09-
van V03.01-	injury (due to)
injury (due to)	cell phone use Y93.C2
cell phone use Y93.C2	fall (from) (off)
fall (from) (off) V00.121-	scooter was moving V00.141-
other accident V00.128-	scooter was not moving W05.1-
unspecified accident V00.128-	other accident V00.148-
S	unspecified accident V00.148-
Scooter (motorized) – see Accident, transport, nontraffic, mobility scooter or Motorcycle. If not motorized, *see* Scooter, nonmotorized	

Note: These codes are for <u>accidental</u> injuries. Do not use if injury due to military or war operations, legal intervention, complication or misadventure.

Land Transport Accidents, Nontraffic – Segway- Skis

ACCIDENTS - Transport
Land – NONTRAFFIC V00-V89

S (continued)
Segway V00.848
collided (with)
animal (being ridden) V06.038
animal drawn vehicle V06.038
bus V04.038
car V03.038
fixed or stationary object V00.842
heavy transport vehicle V04.038
hoverboard (two hoverboards collide) V06.038
motorcycle V02.038
other motor vehicle V06.038
other nonmotor vehicle V06.038
pedal cycle V01.038
pedestrian (on foot or using conveyance) V06.038
pick-up truck V03.038
railway vehicle (train) V05.038
sport utility vehicle V03.038
streetcar (nonpowered) V06.038
three-wheeled vehicle V02.038
truck V04.09-
van V03.038
fell (from) (0ff) V00.848
injury (due to)
cell phone use Y93.C2
fall (from) (off) V00.181-
Skateboard V00.138-
collided (with)
animal being ridden V06.02-
animal-drawn vehicle V06.02-
bus V04.02-
car V03.02-
fixed or stationary object V00.132-
heavy transport vehicle V04.02-
military vehicle V09.01-
motorcycle V02.02-
other land transport vehicle – *see* V01-V09 with 5th character 9
other nonmotor vehicle V06.02-
pedal cycle V01.02-
pedestrian (on foot/using conveyance) V00.02-
pick-up truck V03.02-
railway vehicle (train) V05.02-

S (continued)
Skateboard V00.138- (continued)
collided (with) (continued)
skateboard (two skateboarders collided) V00.138-
sport utility vehicle V03.02-
streetcar (nonpowered) V06.02-
three wheeled vehicle V02.02-
truck V04.02-
van V03.02-
injury (due to)
cell phone use Y93.C2
fall (from) (off) V00.131-
other and unspecified accident V00.138-
Ski lift (any accident) V98.3-
Skis (snow) V00.328-
collided (with)
animal being ridden V06.09-
animal-drawn vehicle V06.09-
bus V04.09-
car V03.09-
fixed or stationary object V00.322-
heavy transport vehicle V04.09-
hoverboard V09.09-
military vehicle V09.01-
motorcycle V02.09-
other motor vehicle V09.0-
other nonmotor vehicle V06.09-
pedal cycle V01.09-
pedestrian (on foot or using conveyance) V00.328-
pick-up truck V03.09-
railway vehicle (train) V05.09-
Segway V09.09-
skis (two skiers collided) V00.328-
sport utility vehicle V03.09-
streetcar (nonpowered) V06.09-
three wheeled vehicle V02.09-
truck V04.09-
van V03.09-
injury (due to)
fall (from) (off) V00.321-
Injury due to cell phone use Y93.C2
other and unspecified accident V00.328-

List intent/cause codes before other External Cause codes. Use more than one code if needed to completely explain the circumstances. **Use these codes throughout treatment with applicable 7th character.**

Land Transport Accidents, Nontraffic – Sled-Standing

ACCIDENTS - Transport
Land – NONTRAFFIC V00-V89

S (continued)
Sled V00.228-
collided (with)
animal being ridden V06.09-
animal-drawn vehicle V06.09-
bus V04.09-
car V03.09-
fixed or stationary object V00.222-
heavy transport vehicle V04.09-
military vehicle V09.01-
motorcycle V02.09-
other land transport vehicle – see V01-V09 with 5th character 9
other nonmotor vehicle V06.09-
pedal cycle V01.09-
pedestrian (on foot or using conveyance) V00.228-
pick-up truck V03.09-
railway vehicle (train) V05.09-
sled (two sleds collide) V00.228-
sport utility vehicle V03.09-
streetcar (nonpowered) V06.09-
three-wheeled vehicle V02.09-
truck V04.09-
van V03.09-
Injury (due to)
cell phone use Y93.C2
fall (from) (off) V00.221-
other and unspecified accident V00.228-
Snowboard V00.318-
collided (with)
animal being ridden V06.09-
animal-drawn vehicle V06.09-
bus V04.09-
car V03.09-
fixed or stationary object V00.312-
heavy transport vehicle V04.09-
military vehicle V09.01-

S (continued)
Snowboard V00.318- (continued)
collided (with) (continued)
motorcycle V02.09-
other land transport vehicle – see V01-V09 with 5th character 9
pedal cycle V01.09-
pedestrian (on foot or using conveyance) V00.318-
pick-up truck V03.09-
railway vehicle (train) V05.09-
sled V00.318-
snowboard (two snowboarders collided) V00.318-
sport utility vehicle V03.09-
streetcar (nonpowered) V06.09-
three-wheeled vehicle V02.09-
truck V04.09-
van V03.09-
Injury (due to)
cell phone use Y93.C2
fall (from) (off) V00.311-
other specified accident V00.318-
unspecified accident V00.318-
Snowmobile V86.92-
injury (due to) (while)
airbag W22.1-
boarding or alighting snowmobile V86.42-
cell phone use Y93.C2
vehicle fire X01.0-
patient was DRIVER V86.52-
patient was HANGER ON V86.72-
patient was OCCUPANT V86.92-
patient was PASSENGER V86.62-
Sport utility vehicle – see Pick-up truck or van
Standing
electric scooter – see electric scooter
micro-mobility pedestrian conveyance – see hoverboard

If military vehicle involved, use code for military vehicle, NOT type of vehicle. For example, patient was driving a snowmobile that hit a military truck. Use code for snowmobile rider hit by military vehicle, not truck.

Land Transport Accidents, Nontraffic – Streetcar-Three wheeled vehicle

ACCIDENTS - Transport
Land – NONTRAFFIC V00-V89

S (continued)	T
Streetcar (powered) (includes cable car, tram, trolley) (includes passenger, conductor, other crew) V82.8-	**Three wheeled vehicle** (motorized) V39.3- – If vehicle not motorized, *see* pedal cycle
collided (with)	patient was DRIVER
animal being ridden V82.8-	collided (with)
animal-drawn vehicle V82.8-	animal V30.0-
bus V82.0-	being ridden V36.0--
car V82.0-	animal-drawn vehicle V36.0-
fixed of stationary object V82.3-	bus V34.0-
heavy transport vehicle V82.0--	car V33.0-
hoverboard V82.0-	fixed or stationary object V37.0-
military vehicle V82.8-	heavy transport vehicle V34.0-
motorcycle V82.0-	hoverboard V39.09-
other motor vehicle V82.0-	military vehicle V39.81-
other nonmotor vehicle V82.8-	motorcycle V32.0-
other object V82.3-	motor vehicle NEC V39.09-
railway vehicle (train) V82.8-	motor vehicle NOS V39.00-
rolling stock V82.2-	other nonmotor vehicle V36.0-
Segway V82.0-	pedal cycle V31.0-
streetcar (two streetcars collided) V82.8-	pedestrian (on foot or using conveyance) V30.0-
three-wheeled vehicle V82.0-	pick-up truck V33.0-
truck V82.0-	railway vehicle (train) V35.0-
van V82.0-	Segway V39.09-
injury (due to) (while)	sport utility vehicle V33.0-
boarding or alighting streetcar V82.4-	streetcar V36.0-
cell phone use Y93.C2	three-wheeled motor vehicle (2 three-wheeled vehicles collided) V32.0-
derailment of streetcar	
without collision V82.7-	truck V34.0-
fall after derailment V82.0-	van V33.0-
fall following collision V82.0-	injury (due to) (while)
fall V82.5-	airbag W22.11-
with derailment V82.0-	boarding or alighting vehicle – *see* Accident, transport, nontraffic, three-wheeled vehicle, occupant
fall *from* streetcar V82.6-	
fall *in* streetcar V82.5-	cell phone use Y93.C2
following collision V82.0-	vehicle fire X01.0-
vehicle fire X01.0-	noncollision accident V38.0-
other specified accident V82.8-	other specified accident V39.89-
unspecified accident V82.9-	

These codes are for accidental injuries. Do not use if injury is due to military or war operations, legal intervention or medical treatment/complication.

List intent/cause codes before other External Cause codes. Use more than one code if needed to completely explain the circumstances. **Use these codes throughout treatment with applicable 7th character.**

If military vehicle involved, use code for military vehicle, NOT type of vehicle. For example, patient driving three wheeled vehicle collided with military truck. Use code for driver of three wheeled vehicle collided with military vehicle, not with truck.

©2020 Terry Tropin. All Rights Reserved.

Land Transport Accidents, Nontraffic – Three wheeled vehicle (continued)

ACCIDENTS - Transport
Land – NONTRAFFIC V00-V89

T (continued)
three wheeled vehicle (motorized) V39.3- – If vehicle not motorized, *see* pedal cycle
patient was HANGER-ON
collided (with)
animal V30.2-
being ridden V36.2-
animal-drawn vehicle V36.2-
bus V34.2-
car V33.2-
fixed or stationary object V37.2-
heavy transport vehicle V34.2-
hoverboard V39.29-
military vehicle 39.81-
motorcycle V32.2-
motor vehicle NEC V39.29-
motor vehicle NOS V39.20-
other nonmotor vehicle V36.2-
pedal cycle V31.2-
pedestrian (on foot/using conveyance) V30.2-
pick-up truck V33.2-
railway vehicle (train) V35.2-
Segway V39.29-
sport utility vehicle V33.2-
streetcar V36.2-
three-wheeled motor vehicle (2 three-wheeled vehicles collided) V32.2-
truck V34.2-
van V33.2-
injury (due to) (while)
boarding or alighting vehicle – *see* Accident, transport, nontraffic, three-wheeled vehicle, Occupant
vehicle fire X01.0-
noncollision accident V38.2-
other specified accident V39.89-
unspecified accident V39.3-
patient was OCCUPANT
collided (with)
animal V30.3-
being ridden V36.3-
animal-drawn vehicle V36.3-
bus V34.3-
car V33.3-
fixed or stationary object V37.3-
heavy transport vehicle V34.3-
hoverboard V39.2-

T (continued)
three wheeled vehicle (motorized) V39.3- (continued) – If vehicle not motorized, *see* pedal cycle
patient was OCCUPANT (continued)
collided (with) (continued)
military vehicle V39.81-
motorcycle V32.3-
other motor vehicle V39.2-
other nonmotor vehicle V36.3-
pedal cycle V31.3-
pedestrian (on foot/using conveyance) V30.3-
pick-up truck V33.3-
railway vehicle (train) V35.3-
Segway V39.2-
sport utility vehicle V33.3-
streetcar V36.3-
three-wheeled motor vehicle (2 three-wheeled vehicles collided) V32.3-
truck V34.3-
van V33.3-
injury (due to) (while)
airbag W22.1-
boarding or alighting vehicle (collided with)
animal V30.4-
being ridden V36.4-
animal-drawn vehicle V36.4-
bus V34.4-
car V33.4-
fixed or stationary object V37.4-
heavy transport vehicle V34.4-
motorcycle V32.4-
other nonmotor vehicle V36.4-
other three-wheeled vehicle V32.4-
pedal cycle V31.4-
pedestrian (on foot/using conveyance V30.4-
pick-up truck V33.4-
railway vehicle (train) V35.4-
sport utility vehicle V33.4-
streetcar V36.4-
truck V34.4-
van V33.4-
vehicle fire X01.0-
noncollision accident V38.3-
boarding or alighting vehicle V38.4-
other specified accident V39.89-
unspecified accident V39.3-

ACCIDENTS - Transport
Land – NONTRAFFIC V00-V89

T (continued)
Three wheeled vehicle (motorized) V39.3- – If vehicle not motorized, see pedal cycle (continued)
patient was PASSENGER
collided (with)
animal V30.1-
being ridden V36.1-
animal-drawn vehicle V36.1-
bus V34.1-
car V33.1-
fixed or stationary object V37.1-
heavy transport vehicle V34.1-
hoverboard V39.1-
military vehicle V39.81-
motorcycle V32.1-
other motor vehicle V39.1-
other nonmotor vehicle V36.1-
pedal cycle V31.1-
pedestrian (on foot/using conveyance) V30.1-
pick-up truck V33.1-
railway vehicle (train) V35.1-
Segway V39.1-
streetcar V36.1-
three-wheeled motor vehicle (2 three-wheeled vehicles collided) V32.1-
truck V34.1-
van V33.1-
injury (due to) (while)
airbag W22.12-
boarding or alighting – see Accident, transport, nontraffic, three-wheeled vehicle, occupant
vehicle fire X01.0-
noncollision accident V38.1-
other specified accident V39.89-
unspecified accident V39.3-
Tractor (and trailer) – see Accident, transport, nontraffic, agricultural vehicle
Train—see Accident, transport, nontraffic, railway vehicle
Tram —see Accident, transport, nontraffic, streetcar
in mine or quarry – see Accident, transport, industrial Vehicle
Tricycle–see Accident, transport, traffic, pedal cycle
motorized – see Accident, transport, nontraffic, three-wheeled vehicle
Trolley – see Accident, transport, nontraffic, streetcar

T (continued)
Truck (18-wheeler, armored or paneled truck, transport vehicle) V69.3- - see also pick-up truck or van
patient was DRIVER
collided (with)
animal V60.0-
being ridden V66.0-
animal-drawn vehicle V66.0-
bus V64.0-
car V63.0-
fixed or stationary object V67.0-
heavy transport vehicle V64.0-
hoverboard V69.09-
military vehicle V69.81-
motorcycle V62.0-
motor vehicle NEC V69.09-
motor vehicle NOS V69.00-
other nonmotor vehicle V66.0-
pedal cycle V61.0-
pedestrian (on foot/using conveyance) V60.0-
pick-up truck V63.0-
railway vehicle (train) V65.0-
Segway V69.09-
sport utility vehicle V63.0-
streetcar V66.0-
three-wheeled motor vehicle V62.0-
truck (two trucks collided) V64.0-
van V63.0-
injury (due to) (while)
airbag W22.11-
boarding or alighting truck – see Accident, transport, nontraffic, truck, occupant
cell phone use Y93.C2
vehicle fire X01.0-
noncollision accident V68.5-
other specified accidents NEC V69.88-
unspecified accident V69.3-

These codes are used for <u>accidental</u> injuries. Do not use if injury is due to military or war operations, legal intervention or medical treatment/complication.

List intent/cause codes before other External Cause codes. Use more than one code if needed to completely explain the circumstances. **Use these codes throughout treatment with applicable 7th character.**

ACCIDENTS - Transport
Land – NONTRAFFIC V00-V89

T (continued)
Truck (18-wheeler, armored or paneled truck, heavy transport vehicle) V69.3- (continued) - see also pick-up truck or van
patient was HANGER-ON
collided (with)
animal V60.2-
being ridden V66.2-
animal-drawn vehicle V66.2-
bus V64.2-
car V63.2-
fixed or stationary object V67.2-
heavy transport vehicle V64.2-
hoverboard V69.29-
military vehicle V69.81-
motorcycle V62.2-
motor vehicle NEC V69.29-
motor vehicle NOS V69.20-
other nonmotor vehicle V66.2-
pedal cycle V61.2-
pedestrian (on foot or using conveyance) V60.2-
pick-up truck V63.2-
railway vehicle (train) V65.2-
Segway V69.29-
sport utility vehicle V63.2-
streetcar V66.2-
three-wheeled motor vehicle V62.2-
truck (two trucks collided) V64.2-
van V63.2-
injury (due to) (while)
boarding or alighting truck – *see* Accident, transport, nontraffic, truck, occupant
vehicle fire X01.0-
noncollision accident V68.2-
other specified accidents V69.88-
unspecified accidents V69.3-
patient was OCCUPANT
collided (with)
animal V60.3-
being ridden V66.3-
animal-drawn vehicle V66.3-
bus V64.3-
car V63.3-
fixed or stationary object V67.3-
heavy transport vehicle V64.3-
hoverboard V69.2-

T (continued)
Truck (18-wheeler, armored or paneled truck, heavy transport vehicle) V69.3- (continued) - see also pick-up truck or van
patient was OCCUPANT (continued)
collided (with) (continued)
military vehicle V69.81-
motorcycle V62.3-
other motor vehicle V69.2-
other nonmotor vehicle V66.3-
pedal cycle V61.3-
pedestrian (on foot/using conveyance) V60.3-
pick-up truck V63.3-
railway vehicle (train) V65.3-
Segway V69.2-
sport utility vehicle V63.3-
streetcar V66.3-
three-wheeled motor vehicle V62.3-
truck (2 trucks collided) V64.3-
van V63.3-
injury (due to) (while)
airbag W22.1-
boarding or alighting truck (collided with)
animal V60.4-
being ridden V66.4-
animal-drawn vehicle V66.4-
bus V64.4-
car V63.4-
fixed or stationary object V67.4-
heavy transport vehicle V64.4-
motorcycle V62.4-
other nonmotor vehicle V66.4-
pedal cycle V61.4-
pedestrian (on foot) V60.4-
pick-up truck V63.4-
railway vehicle (train) V65.4-
sport utility vehicle V63.4-
streetcar V66.4-
three-wheeled vehicle V62.4-
truck V64.4-
van V63.4-
vehicle fire X01.0-
noncollision accident V68.3-
while boarding or alighting V68.4-
other specified accident V69.88-
unspecified accident V69.3-

If military vehicle involved, use code for military vehicle, NOT type of vehicle. For example, patient was driving truck that hit military vehicle. Use code for truck driver collided with military vehicle, not truck.

©2020 Terry Tropin. All Rights Reserved.

ACCIDENTS - Transport
Land – NONTRAFFIC V00-V89

T (continued)
Truck (18-wheeler, armored or paneled truck, heavy transport vehicle) V69.3- (continued)- *see also* Pick-up truck or van
patient was PASSENGER
collided (with)
animal V60.1-
being ridden V66.1-
animal-drawn vehicle V66.1-
bus V64.1-
car V63.1-
fixed or stationary object V67.1-
heavy transport vehicle V64.1-
hoverboard V69.1-
military vehicle V69.81-
motorcycle V62.1-
other motor vehicle V69.1-
other nonmotor vehicle V66.1-
pedal cycle V61.1-
pedestrian (on foot/using conveyance) V60.1-
pick-up truck V63.1-
railway vehicle (train) V65.1-
Segway V69.1-
sport utility vehicle V63.1-
streetcar V66.1-
three-wheeled motor vehicle V62.1-
truck (2 trucks collided) V64.1-
van V63.1-
injury (due to) (while)
airbag W22.12-
boarding or alighting truck –*see* Accident transport, nontraffic, truck, occupant
vehicle fire X01.0-
noncollision accident V68.1-
other specified accidents NEC V69.88-
unspecified accident V69.3-
Two-wheeled vehicle (motorized) – *see* Accident, transport, nontraffic, motorcycle. If not motorized, see pedal cycle

List intent/cause codes before other External Cause codes. Use more than one code if needed to completely explain the circumstances. **Use these codes throughout treatment with applicable 7th character.**

These codes are for <u>accidental</u> injuries. Do not use if accident is due to military or war operations, legal intervention or medical treatment/complications.

U
Unknown vehicle (vehicles involved in accident known but not which vehicle was patient's) V89.9-
collision involved
bus and
car V88.3-
heavy transport vehicle V88.5-
motorcycle V88.1-
pick-up truck V88.7-
three-wheeled vehicle V88.1-
van V88.2
car and
bus V88.3-
heavy transport vehicle V88.4-
motorcycle V88.0-
pick-up truck V88.2-
railway vehicle (train) V88.6-
three-wheeled motor vehicle V88.0-
van V88.2-
heavy transport vehicle and
bus V88.5-
car V88.4-
motorcycle and
bus V88.3-
car V88.0-
three-wheeled vehicle V88.1-
other motor vehicle and
motorcycle V88.1-
three-wheeled vehicle V88.1-
pick-up truck and
bus V88.7-
car V88.2-
railway vehicle (train) and
car V88.6-
three-wheeled vehicle and
bus V88.1-
car V88.0-
van and
bus V88.2-
car V88.2-
noncollision accident involving
other motor vehicles V88.8-
other nonmotor vehicles V88.9-
other accident involving
other motor vehicle V88.7-
other nonmotor vehicle V88.9-
pedal cycle – *see* V10-V19
pedestrian – *see* V01-V09

Land Transport Accidents, Nontraffic – Van-Wheeled shoes

ACCIDENTS - Transport
Land – NONTRAFFIC V00-V89

V
Van – see Pick-up truck
W
Walking – see Pedestrian (on foot or using conveyance)
Wheelchair (powered) V00.818-
collided (with)
animal being ridden V06.09-
animal drawn vehicle V06.09-
bus V04.09-
car V03.09-
fixed or stationary object V00.812-
heavy transport vehicle V04.09-
hoverboard V09.0-
military vehicle V09.01-
motorcycle V02.09-
other motor vehicle V09.0-
other nonmotor vehicle V06.09-
pedal cycle V01.09-
pedestrian (on foot or using conveyance) V00.09-
pick-up truck V03.09-
railway vehicle (train) V05.09-
Segway V09.0=
sport utility vehicle V03.09-
streetcar (nonpowered) V06.09-
three-wheeled vehicle V02.09-
truck V04.09-
van V03.09-
wheelchair (two wheelchairs collided) V00.818-
injury (due to) (while)
boarding or alighting wheelchair V00.818-
cell phone use Y93.C2
fall (from) (out)
wheelchair was moving V00.811-
wheelchair was not moving W05.0-
noncollision accident V00.818-
other accident V00.818-
unspecified accident V00.818-
Wheeled shoes – see Heelies

If military vehicle involved, use code for military vehicle, NOT type of vehicle. For example, patient was in wheelchair hit by military truck. Use code for pedestrian collided with. military vehicle, not truck

END OF ACCIDENT, TRANSPORT, LAND, NONTRAFFIC

ACCIDENTS - Transport
Land – TRAFFIC V00-V89

A

Agriculture vehicle (includes farm machinery, tractor, harvester, trailer) V84.3- (Excludes animal-powered vehicle)
- injury (due to) (while)
  - airbag W22.1-
  - boarding or alighting vehicle V84.4-
  - cell phone use Y93.C2
  - vehicle fire X01.0-
  - vehicle stationary or in maintenance W30.81-
- patient was DRIVER V84.0-
- patient was HANGER-ON V84.2-
- patient was OCCUPANT V84.3-
- patient was PASSENGER V84.1

All-terrain vehicle (includes go cart, golf cart or off-road vehicle) V86.3- see also specific vehicle
- injury (due to) (while)
  - airbag W22.1-
  - boarding or alighting vehicle V86.45-
  - cell phone use Y93.C2
  - vehicle fire X01.0-
  - vehicle stationary or in maintenance W31.81-
- patient was DRIVER V86.05-
- patient was HANGER-ON V86.25-
- patient was OCCUPANT V86.35-
- patient was PASSENGER V86.15-

Ambulance V86.39-
- injury (due to) (while)
  - airbag W22.1-
  - boarding or alighting ambulance V86.41-
  - cell phone use Y93.C2
  - vehicle fire X01.0-
  - vehicle stationary or in maintenance W31-
- patient was DRIVER V86.01-
- patient was HANGER-ON V86.21-
- patient was OCCUPANT V86.31-
- patient was PASSENGER V86.11-

Animal-drawn vehicle (includes horse-drawn carriage, donkey-carts, dogsleds) V80.929-
- collided (with)
  - animal V80.12-
    - being ridden V80.711-
  - animal-drawn vehicle (two animal-drawn vehicles collided) V80.721-
  - bus V80.42-
  - car V80.42-
  - fixed or stationary object V80.82-
  - heavy transport vehicle V80.42-
  - hoverboard V80.52-
  - military vehicle V80.920-
  - motorcycle V80.32-
  - other motor vehicle V80.52-
  - other nonmotor vehicle V80.791-
  - pedal cycle V80.22-
  - pedestrian (on foot or using conveyance) V80.12-
  - pick-up truck V80.42-
  - railway vehicle (train) V80.62-
  - Segway V80.52-
  - sport utility vehicle V80.42-
  - streetcar V80.731-
  - three-wheeled motor vehicle V80.32-
  - truck V80.42-
  - van V80.42-
- injury (due to) (while)
  - cell phone use Y93.C2
  - vehicle fire X01.0-
- noncollision accident V80.02-
- other accident V80.928-
- unspecified accident V80.929-

These codes are used for <u>accidental</u> injuries. Do not use if injury is due to military or war operations, legal interventions Or medical treatment/complication/

Land Transport Accidents, Traffic – Animal-rider-Bulldozer

ACCIDENTS - Transport
Land – TRAFFIC V00-V89

A	B
Animal-rider (any animal) V80.919-	**Baby stroller** (patient pushing or in stroller) V00.828-
collided (with)	collided (with)
animal V80.11-	animal V06.19-
being ridden (2 riders collided) V80.710-	being ridden V06.19-
animal-drawn vehicle V80.720-	animal-drawn vehicle V06.19-
bus V80.41-	baby stroller (2 strollers collided) V06.19-
car V80.41-	bus V04.19-
fixed or stationary object V80.81-	car V03.19-
heavy transport vehicle V80.41-	fixed or stationary object V00.822-
hoverboard V80.51-	heavy transport vehicle V04.19-
military vehicle V80.910-	hoverboard V09.19-
motorcycle V80.31-	military vehicle V09.21-
other motor vehicle V80.51-	motorcycle V02.19-
other nonmotor vehicle V80.790-	motor vehicle NEC V09.19-
pedal cycle V80.21-	motor vehicle NOS V09.10-
pedestrian (on foot or using conveyance) V80.11-	other nonmotor vehicle V06.19-
pick-up truck V80.41-	pedal cycle V01.19-
railway vehicle (train) V80.61-	pedestrian (on foot/using conveyance) V06.19-
Segway V80.51-	pick-up truck V03.19-
sport utility vehicle V80.41-	railway vehicle (train) V05.19-
streetcar V80.730-	sport utility vehicle V03.19-
three-wheeled motor vehicle V80.31-	streetcar (nonpowered) V06.19-
truck V80.41-	three-wheeled motor vehicle V02.19-
van V80.41-	truck V04.19-
noncollision accident	van V03.19-
patient was riding horse V80.010-	Injury cell phone use Y93.C2
patient was riding other animal V80.018-	noncollision accident (fall from stroller) V00.821-
other accident V80.918-	other specified accident V00.828-
unspecified accident V80.929-	unspecified accident V00.828-
Armored car —see Accident, transport, traffic, truck	**Battery-powered truck** (baggage) – see Accident, transport, traffic, Industrial vehicle
	Bicycle –see Accident, transport, traffic, pedal cycle
	Bulldozer – see Accident, transport, traffic, construction

List intent/cause codes before other External Cause Codes. Use more than one code if needed to completely explain the circumstances. **Use these codes throughout treatment with applicable 7th character.**

ACCIDENTS - Transport
Land – TRAFFIC V00-V89

B (continued)

Bus (includes motor coach) V79.9-
- patient was DRIVER
  - collided (with)
    - animal V70.5-
      - being ridden V76.5-
    - animal-drawn vehicle V76.5-
    - bus (two buses collided) V74.5-
    - car V73.5-
    - fixed or stationary object V77.5-
    - heavy transport vehicle V74.5-
    - hoverboard V79.49-
    - military vehicle V79.81-
    - motorcycle V72.5-
    - motor vehicle NEC V79.49-
    - motor vehicle NOS V79.40-
    - other nonmotor vehicle V76.5-
    - pedal cycle V71.5-
    - pedestrian (on foot/using conveyance) V70.5-
    - pick-up truck V73.5-
    - railway vehicle (train) V75.5-
    - Segway V79.49-
    - sport utility vehicle V73.5-
    - streetcar (nonpowered) V76.5-
    - three-wheeled motor vehicle V72.5-
    - truck V74.5-
    - van V73.5-
  - injury (due to) (while)
    - airbag W22.11-
    - boarding or alighting bus – see Accident, transport, traffic, bus, occupant
    - cell phone use Y93.C2
    - vehicle fire X01.0-
  - noncollision accident V78.5-
  - other specified accident V79.88-
  - unspecified accident V79.9-

Bus (includes motor coach) V79.9- (continued)
- patient was HANGER-ON
  - collided (with)
    - animal V70.7-
      - being ridden V76.7-
    - animal-drawn vehicle V76.7-
    - bus (two buses collided) V74.7-
    - car V73.7-
    - fixed or stationary object V77.7-
    - heavy transport vehicle V74.7-
    - hoverboard V79.49-
    - military vehicle V79.81-
    - motorcycle V72.7-
    - motor vehicle NEC V79.49-
    - motor vehicle NOS V79.40-
    - other nonmotor vehicle V76.7-
    - pedal cycle V71.7-
    - pedestrian (on foot/using conveyance) V70.7-
    - pick-up truck V73.7-
    - railway vehicle (train) V75.7-
    - Segway V79.49-
    - sport utility vehicle V73.7-
    - streetcar (nonpowered) V76.7-
    - three wheeled motor vehicle V72.7-
    - truck V74.7-
    - van V73.7-
  - injury (due to) (while)
    - boarding or alighting bus – see Accident, transport, traffic, bus, occupant
    - vehicle fire X01.0-
  - noncollision accident V78.7-
  - other specified accident V79.88-
  - unspecified accident V79.9-

If military vehicle involved, use code for military vehicle, **NOT** type of vehicle. For example, bus driver collided with military motorcycle. Use code for bus driver collied with military vehicle, not bus driver collided with motorcycle.

ACCIDENTS - Transport
Land – TRAFFIC V00-V89

B (continued)

Bus (includes motor coach) (continued) V79.6-	**Bus** (motor coach) (continued) V79.9-
patient was OCCUPANT V79.9-	patient was OCCUPANT (continued)
collided (with)	noncollision accident V78.9-
animal V70.9-	other specified accident V79.88-
being ridden V76.9-	unspecified accident V79.9-
animal-drawn vehicle V76.9-	patient was PASSENGER
bus (two buses collided) V74.9-	collided (with)
car V73.9-	animal V70.6-
fixed or stationary object V77.9-	being ridden V76.6-
heavy transport vehicle V74.9-	animal-drawn vehicle V76.6-
hoverboard V79.69-	bus (two buses collided) V74.6-
military vehicle V79.81-	car V73.6-
motorcycle V72.9-	fixed or stationary object V77.6-
motor vehicle NEC V79.69-	heavy transport vehicle V74.6-
motor vehicle NOS V79.60-	hoverboard V79.59-
other nonmotor vehicle V76.9-	military vehicle V79.81-
pedal cycle V71.9-	motorcycle V72.6-
pedestrian (on foot/using conveyance) V70.9-	motor vehicle NEC V79.59-
pick-up truck V73.9-	motor vehicle NOS V79.50-
railway vehicle (train) V75.9-	other nonmotor vehicle V76.6-
Segway V79.69-	pedal cycle V71.6-
sport utility vehicle V73.9-	pedestrian (on foot/using conveyance) V70.6-
streetcar V76.9-	pick-up truck V73.6-
three wheeled motor vehicle V72.9-	railway vehicle V75.6-
truck V74.9-	Segway V79.49-
van V73.9-	sport utility vehicle V73.6-
injury (due to) (while)	streetcar (nonpowered) V76.6-
airbag W22.1-	three wheeled motor vehicle V72.6-
boarding or alighting (collided with)	truck V74.6-
animal V70.4-	van V73.6-
being ridden V76.4-	injury (due to) (while)
animal-drawn vehicle V76.4-	airbag W22.1-
bus V74.4-	boarding or alighting bus– *see* Accident, transport, traffic, bus, occupant
car V73.4-	vehicle fire X01.0-
fixed or stationary object V77.4-	noncollision accident V78.6-
heavy transport vehicle V74.4-	other specified accident V79.59-
motorcycle V72.4-	unspecified accident V79.50-
other nonmotor vehicle V76.4-	
pedal cycle V71.4-	
pedestrian (on foot/using conveyance) V70.4-	
pick-up truck V73.4-	
railway vehicle (train) V75.4-	
sport utility vehicle V73.4-	
streetcar V76.4-	
three-wheeled vehicle V72.4-	
truck V74.4-	
van V73.4-	
vehicle fire X01.0-	

These codes are for <u>accidental</u> injuries. Do not use if accident is due to military or war operations, legal intervention or medical treatment/complication.

Land Transport Accidents, Traffic – Cable car-Car

ACCIDENTS - Transport
Land – TRAFFIC V00-V89

C
Cable car, not on rails V98.0-
on rails —*see* Accident, transport, traffic, streetcar
Car V49.60-
patient was DRIVER
collided (with)
animal V40.5-
being ridden V46.5-
animal-drawn vehicle V46.5-
bus V44.5-
car (two cars collided) V43.52-
fixed or stationary object V47.5-
heavy transport vehicle V44.5-
hoverboard V49.49-
military vehicle V49.81-
motorcycle V42.5-
motor vehicle NEC V49.49-
motor vehicle NOS V49.40-
other nonmotor vehicle V46.5-
pedal cycle V41.5-
pedestrian (on foot/using conveyance) V40.5-
pick-up truck V43.53-
railway vehicle (train) V45.5-
Segway V49.49-
sport utility vehicle V43.51-
streetcar (nonpowered) V46.5-
three wheeled motor vehicle V42.5-
truck V44.5-
van V43.54-
injury (due to) (while)
airbag W22.11-
boarding or alighting bus – *see* Accident, transport, traffic, car, occupant
cell phone use Y93.C2
vehicle fire X01.0-
noncollision accident V48.5-
other specified accidents V49.49-
unspecified accidents V49.40-

C (continued)
Car V49.60- (continued)
patient was HANGER-ON
collided (with)
animal V40.7-
being ridden V46.7-
animal-drawn vehicle V46.7-
bus V44.7-
car (two cars collided) V43.72-
fixed or stationary object V47.7-
heavy transport vehicle V44.7-
hoverboard V49.69-
military vehicle V49.81-
motorcycle V42.7-
motor vehicle NEC V49.69-
motor vehicle NOS V49.60-
other nonmotor vehicle V46.7-
pedal cycle V41.7-
pedestrian (on foot/using conveyance) V40.7
pick-up truck V43.73-
railway vehicle (train) V45.7-
Segway V49.69-
sport utility vehicle V43.71-
streetcar (nonpowered) V46.7-
three wheeled motor vehicle V42.7-
truck V44.7-
van V43.74-
injury (due to) (while)
boarding or alighting – *see* Accident, transport, traffic, car, occupant
vehicle fire X01.0-
noncollision accident V48.7-
other specified accidents V49.69-
unspecified accidents V49.60-

List intent/cause codes before other External Cause codes. Use more than one code if needed to completely explain the circumstances. **Use these codes throughout treatment with applicable 7th character.**

ACCIDENTS - Transport
Land – TRAFFIC V00-V89

C (continued)

Car V49.60- (continued)
- patient was OCCUPANT
  - collided (with)
    - animal V40.9-
      - being ridden V46.9-
    - animal-drawn vehicle V46.9-
    - bus V44.9-
    - car (two cars collided) V43.92-
    - fixed or stationary object V47.9-
    - heavy transport vehicle V44.9-
    - hoverboard V49.69-
    - military vehicle V49.81-
    - motorcycle V42.9-
    - motor vehicle NEC V49.69-
    - motor vehicle NOS V49.60-
    - other nonmotor vehicle V46.69-
    - pedal cycle V41.9-
    - pedestrian (on foot/using conveyance) V40.9-
    - pick-up truck V43.93-
    - railway vehicle (train) V45.9-
    - Segway V49.69-
    - sport utility vehicle V43.91-
    - streetcar (nonpowered) V46.9-
    - three wheeled motor vehicle V42.9-
    - truck V44.9-
    - van V43.94-
  - injury (due to) (while)
    - airbag W22.1-
    - boarding or alighting car (collided with) V48.4-
      - animal V40.4-
        - being ridden V46.4-
      - animal-drawn vehicle V46.4-
      - bus V44.4-
      - car (two cars collided) V43.42-
      - fixed or stationary object V47.4-
      - heavy transport vehicle V44.4-
      - motorcycle V42.4-
      - other nonmotor vehicle V46.4-
      - pedal cycle V41.4-
      - pedestrian (on foot/using conveyance) V40.4-
      - pick-up truck V43.43-
      - railway vehicle (train) V45.4-
      - sport utility vehicle V43.41-
      - streetcar V46.4-
      - three-wheeled vehicle V42.4-
      - truck V44.4-
      - van V43.44-
    - vehicle fire X01.0-

C (continued)

Car V49.9- (continued)
- patient was OCCUPANT (continued)
  - noncollision accident V48.9-
    - while boarding or alighting car V48.4-
  - other specified accidents V49.69-
  - unspecified accidents V49.60-
- patient was PASSENGER
  - collided (with)
    - animal V40.6-
      - being ridden V46.6-
    - animal-drawn vehicle V46.6-
    - bus V44.6-
    - car (two cars collided) V43.62-
    - fixed or stationary object V47.6-
    - heavy transport vehicle V44.6-
    - hoverboard V49.59-
    - military vehicle V49.81-
    - motorcycle V42.6-
    - motor vehicle NEC V49.59-
    - motor vehicle NOS V49.50-
    - other nonmotor vehicle V46.6-
    - pedal cycle V41.6-
    - pedestrian (on foot/using conveyance) V40.6-
    - pick-up truck V43.63-
    - railway vehicle (train) V45.6-
    - Segway V49.59-
    - sport utility vehicle V43.61-
    - streetcar V46.59-
    - three wheeled motor vehicle V42.6-
    - truck V44.6-
    - van V43.64-
  - injury (due to) (while)
    - airbag W22.10-
    - boarding or alighting – *see* Accident, transport, traffic, car, occupant
    - cell phone use Y93.C2
    - vehicle fire X01.0-
  - noncollision accident V48.6-
  - other specified accident V49.88-
  - unspecified accident V49.9-

If military vehicle involved, use code for military vehicle **NOT** Type of vehicle. For example, patient was driving a car that collided with military truck. Use code for driver collided with military vehicle, not driver collided with truck.

ACCIDENTS - Transport
Land – TRAFFIC V00-V89

C (continued)
Coal car - *see* Accident, transport, traffic, industrial vehicle
Construction vehicle (includes bulldozer, digger, dump truck, earth leveler, mechanical shovel)
injury (due to) (while)
airbag W22.19-
boarding or alighting vehicle V85.4-
cell phone use Y93.C2
vehicle fire X01.0-
vehicle stationary or in maintenance W31-
patient was DRIVER V85.0-
patient was HANGER-ON V85.2-
patient was OCCUPANT V85.3-
patient was PASSENGER V85.1-
D
Digger – *see* Accident, transport, traffic, construction vehicle
Dirt bike – (includes motor/cross bike) - *see also* Accident, transport, traffic, all-terrain
injury (due to) (while)
boarding or alighting V86.46-
cell phone use Y93.C2
vehicle fire X01.0-
vehicle stationary or in maintenance W31-
patient was DRIVER V86.06-
patient was HANGER ON V86.26-
patient was OCCUPANT V86.36-
patient was PASSENGER V86.16-
Dump truck – *see* Accident, transport, traffic, construction vehicle
Dune buggy
injury (due to) (while)
boarding or alighting dune buggy V86.43-
cell phone use Y93.C2
vehicle fire X01.0-
patient was DRIVER V86.03-
patient was HANGER ON V86.23-
patient was OCCUPANT V86.33-
patient was PASSENGER V86.13-

E
Earth-leveler – see Accident, transport, traffic, construction vehicle
Electric scooter (standing) – see also Hoverboard
collision (with)
animal (being ridden) V06.131
animal drawn vehicle V06.131
bus V04.131
car V03.131
electric scooter (two scooters collide) V06.131
fixed or stationary object V00.842
heavy transport vehicle V04.131
hoverboard V06.131
motorcycle V02.131
other motor vehicle V06.131
other nonmotor vehicle V06.131
other nonmotor vehicle V06.131
pedal cycle V01.131
pedestrian (on foot/using conveyance) V06.131
pick-up truck V03.131
railway vehicle (train) V05.131
sport utility vehicle V03.131
streetcar (nonpowered) V06.131
three-wheeled vehicle V02.131
truck V04.19-
van V03.131
fell (from) off) V00.841
Injury due to cell phone use Y93.C2

These codes are used for <u>accidental</u> injuries. Do not use If injury is due to military or war operations, legal Intervention, or medical treatment/complication.

Land Transport Accidents, Traffic – Farm machinery-Hoverboard

ACCIDENTS - Transport
Land – TRAFFIC V00-V89

F	
Farm machinery – see Accident, transport, traffic, agricultural vehicle	
Fire engine (truck) V86.01-	
	injury (due to) (while)
		airbag W22.1-
		boarding or alighting fire engine V86.41-
		cell phone use Y93.C2
		vehicle fire X01.0-
	patient was DRIVER V86.01-
	patient was HANGER-ON V86.21-
	patient was OCCUPANT V86.31-
	patient was PASSENGER V86.11-
Forklift —see Accident, transport, traffic, industrial vehicle	
G	
Go cart —see Accident, transport, traffic, all-terrain vehicle	
Golf cart —see Accident, transport, traffic, all-terrain vehicle	
H	
Harvester – see Accident, transport, traffic, agricultural vehicle	
Heavy transport vehicle —see Accident, transport, traffic, truck	
Heelies V00.158-	
	collided (with)
		fixed or stationary object V00.152-
		other object or vehicle V00.158-
		pedestrian (on foot/using conveyance) V00.158-
	injury due to cell phone use Y93.C2
	fell from (off) heelies V00.151-
	noncollision accident V00.158-

H (continued)	
Hoverboard V00.848	
	collided (with)
		animal (being ridden) V06.138
		animal drawn vehicle V06.138
		bus V04.138
		car V03.138
		fixed or stationary object V00.842
		heavy transport vehicle V04.138
		hoverboard (two hoverboards collide) V06.138
		motorcycle V02.138
		other motor vehicle V06.138
		other nonmotor vehicle V06.138
		pedal cycle V01.138
		pedestrian (on foot or using conveyance) V06.138
		pick-up truck V03.138
		railway vehicle (train) V05.138
		Segway V06.138
		sport utility vehicle V03.138
		streetcar (nonpowered) V06.138
		three-wheeled vehicle V02.138
		truck V04.19-
		van V03.138
	fell (from) (0ff) V00.848
	injury due to cell phone use Y93.C2

.List intent/cause codes before other External Cause codes. Use more than one code if needed to completely explain the circumstances. **Use these codes throughout treatment with applicable 7th character.**

ACCIDENTS - Transport
Land – TRAFFIC V00-V89

I

Ice skates V00.21-
- collided (with)
  - animal V06.19-
    - being ridden V06.19-
  - bus V04.19-
  - car V03.19-
  - fixed or stationary object V00.212-
  - heavy transport vehicle V04.19-
  - ice skates (2 ice skaters collided) V00.218-
  - motorcycle V02.19-
  - other land transport vehicle – see V01-V09
  - other nonmotor vehicle V06.19-
  - pedal cycle V01.19-
  - pedestrian (on foot or using conveyance) V06.19-
  - pick-up truck V03.19-
  - railway vehicle (train) V05.10-
  - sport utility vehicle V03.19-
  - streetcar (nonpowered) V06.19-
  - three-wheeled vehicle V02.19-
  - truck V04.19-
  - van V03.19-
- fell from (off) skates V00.211-

Industrial vehicle (includes battery-powered truck, coal car, forklift, logging car, mine tram) V83.3-
- injury (due to) (while)
  - airbag W22.1-
  - boarding or alighting vehicle V83.4-
  - cell phone use Y93.C2
  - vehicle fire X01.0-
  - vehicle stationary or in maintenance W31-
- patient was DRIVER V83.0-
- patient was HANGER-ON V83.2-
- patient was OCCUPANT NOS V83.3-
- patient was PASSENGER V83.1-

L

logging car —see Accident, transport, traffic, industrial vehicle

If military vehicle involved, use code for military vehicle **NOT** Type of vehicle. For example, patient was riding mobility scooter that collided with military motorcycle. Use code for scooter rider collided with military vehicle, not scooter rider collided with motorcycle.

M

Mechanical shovel – see Accident, transport, traffic, construction vehicle

Military vehicle V86.34-
- injury (due to) (while)
  - airbag W22.1-
  - boarding or alighting vehicle V86.44-
  - Injury due to cell phone use Y93.C2
  - vehicle fire X01.0-
- patient was DRIVER V86.04-
- patient was HANGER ON V86.24-
- patient was OCCUPANT V86.34-
- patient was PASSENGER V86.14-

Mine tram —see Accident, transport, traffic, industrial vehicle

Mini-bus – see Accident, transport, traffic, pick-up truck or van

Mini-van – see Accident, transport, traffic, pick-up truck or van

Mobility scooter (motorized) (driver, passenger, or occupant) V00.838-
- collided (with)
  - bus V04.19-
  - car V03.19-
  - fixed or stationary object V00.832-
  - heavy transport vehicle V04.19-
  - hoverboard V09.19-
  - mobility scooter (2 scooters collided) V00.838-
  - motorcycle V02.19-
  - other motor vehicle V09.19-
  - pedal cycle V01.19-
  - pedestrian (on foot or using conveyance) V00.838-
  - pick-up truck V03.19-
  - railway vehicle (train) V05.19-
  - Segway V09.19-
  - sport utility vehicle V03.19-
  - streetcar (nonpowered) V06.19-
  - three-wheeled motor vehicle V02.19-
  - truck V04.19-
  - van V03.19-
- injury (due to) (while)
  - airbag W22.1-
  - cell phone use Y93.C2
  - fall (from) (out) scooter V00.831-
  - vehicle fire X01.0-
- other mobility scooter accident V00.838-

moped – see Accident, transport, traffic, motorcycle

motor/cross bike - see Dirt bike

motor coach – see Accident, transport, traffic, bus

©2020 Terry Tropin. All Rights Reserved.

Land Transport Accidents, Traffic – Motorcycle

ACCIDENTS - Transport
Land – TRAFFIC V00-V89

M (continued)
Motorcycle (includes motorized scooter, moped) V29.60-
patient was DRIVER
collided (with)
animal V20.4-
being ridden V26.4-
animal-drawn vehicle V26.4-
bus V24.4-
car V23.4-
fixed or stationary object V27.4-
heavy transport vehicle V24.4-
hoverboard V29.4-
military vehicle V29.81-
motorcycle (two motorcycles collided) V22.4-
other motor vehicle V29.4-
other nonmotor vehicle V26.4-
pedal cycle V21.4-
pedestrian (on foot/using conveyance) V20.4-
pick-up truck V23.4-
railway vehicle (train) V25.4-
Segway V29.4-
sport utility vehicle V23.4-
streetcar (nonpowered) V26.4-
three wheeled motor vehicle V22.4-
truck V24.4-
van V23.4-
injury (due to) (while)
boarding or alighting – see Accident, transport, traffic, motorcycle, occupant
cell phone use Y93.C2
vehicle fire X01.0-
noncollision accident V28.4-
other specified accident V29.60-
unspecified accident V29.4-
patient was OCCUPANT
collided (with)
animal V20.9-
being ridden V26.9-
animal-drawn vehicle V26.9-
bus V24.9-
car V23.9-
fixed or stationary object V27.9-
heavy transport vehicle V24.9-
hoverboard V29.69-
military vehicle V29.81-
motorcycle (2 motorcycles collided) V22.9
motor vehicle NEC V29.69-

M (continued)
Motorcycle (includes motorized scooter, moped) V29.60-
patient was OCCUPANT (continued)
collided (with) (continued)
other nonmotor vehicle V26.9-
pedal cycle V21.9-
pedestrian (on foot/using conveyance) V20.9-
pick-up truck V23.9-
railway vehicle (train) V25.9-
Segway V29.69-
sport utility vehicle V23.9-
streetcar (nonpowered) V26.9-
three wheeled motor vehicle V22.9-
truck V24.9-
van V23.9-
injury (due to) (while)
boarding or alighting (collided with)
animal V20.3-
being ridden V26.3-
animal-drawn vehicle V26.3-
bus V24.3-
car V23.3-
fixed or stationary object V27.3-
heavy transport vehicle V24.3-
hoverboard V29.69-
military vehicle V29.81-
motorcycle (two motorcycles collided) V29.69-
other motor vehicle V29.69-
other nonmotor vehicle V26.60-
pedal cycle V21.3-
pedestrian (on foot/using conveyance) V20.3-
pick-up truck V23.3-
railway vehicle (train) V25.3-
sport utility vehicle V23.3-
streetcar (nonpowered) V26.3-
three-wheeled vehicle V22.3-
truck V24.3-
van V23.3-
vehicle fire X01.0-
noncollision accident V28.2-
while boarding or lighting V28.3-
other specified accident V29.69-
unspecified accident V29.60-

These codes are for accidental injuries. Do not use if accident is due to military or war operations, legal intervention or medical treatment/complication.

Land Transport Accidents, Traffic – Motorcycle-Pedal cycle

ACCIDENTS - Transport
Land – TRAFFIC V00-V89

M (continued)		O	
Motorcycle (includes motorized scooter, moped) (cont.) V29.60-		**Off road vehicle** – see All terrain vehicle	
patient was PASSENGER		P	
collided (with)		**Pedal cycle** (includes tricycle, bicycle, rickshaw) V19.9-	
animal V20.5-		patient was DRIVER	
being ridden V26.5-		collided (with)	
animal-drawn vehicle V26.5-		animal V10.4-	
bus V24.5-		being ridden V16.4-	
car V23.5-		animal-drawn vehicle V16.4-	
fixed or stationary object V27.5-		bus V14.4-	
heavy transport vehicle V24.5-		car V13.4-	
hoverboard V29.59-		fixed or stationary object V17.4-	
military vehicle V29.81-		heavy transport vehicle V14.4-	
motorcycle (2 motorcycles collided) V22.5-		hoverboard V19.49-	
motor vehicle NEC V29.59-		military vehicle V19.81-	
motor vehicle NOS V29.50-		motorcycle V12.4-	
other nonmotor vehicle V26.5-		motor vehicle NEC V19.49-	
pedal cycle V21.5-		motor vehicle NOS V19.40-	
pedestrian (on foot/using conveyance) V20.5-		other nonmotor vehicle V16.4-	
pick-up truck V23.5-		pedal cycle (2 cycles collided) V11.4-	
railway vehicle (train) V25.5-		pedestrian (on foot/using conveyance) V10.4-	
Segway V29.59-		pick-up truck V13.4-	
sport utility vehicle V23.5-		railway vehicle (train) V15.4-	
streetcar V26.5-		Segway V19.49-	
three wheeled motor vehicle V22.5-		sport utility vehicle V13.4-	
truck V24.5-		streetcar V16.4-	
van V23.5-		three wheeled motor vehicle V12.4-	
injury (due to) (while)		truck V14.4-	
boarding or alighting – see Accident, transport, traffic, motorcycle, occupant		van V13.4-	
		van V13.4-	
vehicle fire X01.0-		injury (due to) (while)	
noncollision accident V28.5-		boarding or alighting – see Accident, transport, traffic, pedal cycle, occupant	
other specified accident V29.69-		cell phone use Y93.C2	
unspecified V29.61-		noncollision accident V18.4-	
Motor vehicle NOS V89.2-		other specified accident V19.198-	
N		unspecified accident V19.40-	
nonmotor vehicle NOS V89.3-			

List intent/cause codes before other External Cause codes. Use more than one code if needed to completely explain the circumstances. **Use these codes throughout treatment with applicable 7th character**.

©2020 Terry Tropin. All Rights Reserved.

Land Transport Accidents, Traffic – Pedal cycle

ACCIDENTS - Transport
Land – TRAFFIC V00-V89

P (continued)
Pedal cycle (includes tricycle, bicycle, rickshaw) (cont). V19.9-
patient was OCCUPANT
collided (with)
animal V10.9-
animal-drawn vehicle V16.9-
bus V14.9-
car V13.9-
fixed or stationary object V17.9-
heavy transport vehicle V14.9-
hoverboard V19.6-
military vehicle V19.81-
motorcycle V12.9-
other motor vehicle V19.6-
other nonmotor vehicle V16.9-
pedal cycle (2 cycles collided) V11.9-
pedestrian (on foot or using conveyance) V10.9-
pick-up truck V13.9-
railway vehicle (train) V15.9-
Segway V14.6-
sport utility vehicle V13.9-
streetcar V16.9-
three wheeled motor vehicle V12.9-
truck V14.9-
van V13.9-
injury (while)
boarding or alighting (collided with)
animal V10.3-
being ridden V16.3-
animal-drawn vehicle V16.3-
bus V14.3-
car V13.3-
fixed or stationary object V17.3-
heavy transport vehicle V14.3-
motorcycle V12.3-
other nonmotor vehicle V16.3-
pedal cycle (2 cycles collided) V11.3-
pedestrian (on foot) V10.3-
pick-up truck V13.3-
railway vehicle (train) V15.3-
sport utility vehicle V13.3-
streetcar V16.3-
three-wheeled vehicle V12.3-
truck V14.3-
van V13.3-

P (continued)
Pedal cycle (includes tricycle, bicycle, rickshaw) (cont.) V19.9-
patient was OCCUPANT (continued)
noncollision accident V18.9-
entanglement in wheel V19.88-
explosion of bicycle tire W37.0-
while boarding or alighting cycle V18.3-
other specified accident V19.88-
unspecified accident V19.9-
patient was PASSENGER
collided (with)
animal V10.5-
animal-drawn vehicle V16.5-
bus V14.5-
car V13.5
fixed or stationary object V17.5-
heavy transport vehicle V14.5-
military vehicle V19.81-
motorcycle V12.5-
other motor vehicle V19.5-
other nonmotor vehicle V16.5-
pedal cycle (two cycles collided) V11.5-
pedestrian (on foot/using conveyance) V10.5-
pick-up truck V13.5
railway vehicle (train) V15.5-
sport utility vehicle V13.1-
streetcar V16.5-
three wheeled motor vehicle V12.5-
truck V14.5-
van V13.1-
injury (while)
boarding or alighting – *see* Accident, transport, traffic, pedal cycle, occupant
noncollision V18.5-
entanglement in wheel V19.88-
explosion of bicycle tire W37.0-
while boarding or alighting cycle V18.3-
other specified V19.88-
unspecified accident V19.9-

If military vehicle involved, use code for military vehicle, **NOT** type of vehicle. For example, if pedal cyclist collided with military motorcycle, use code for pedal cyclist collided with military vehicle not pedal cyclist collided with motorcycle.

ACCIDENTS - Transport
Land – TRAFFIC V00-V89

P (continued)
Pedestrian (on foot) - *see also* Fall, Slipping
collided (with)
animal – *see* Contact, with, animal, struck by
being ridden V06.10-
animal-drawn vehicle V06.10-
bus V04.10-
car V03.10-
fixed or stationary object – *see* Fall, Striking against, etc.
heavy transport vehicle V04.10-
hoverboard V09.29-
military vehicle V09.21-
motorcycle V02.10-
motor vehicle NEC V09.29-
motor vehicle NOS V09.20-
other nonmotor vehicle V06.10-
pedal cycle V01.10-
pedestrian (two pedestrians collided) (without fall) W51-
with fall W03-
due to ice or snow W00.0-
pick-up truck V03.10-
railway vehicle (train) V05.10-
roller skater V00.11-
Segway V09.29-
skateboarder V00.02-
sport utility vehicle V03.10-
streetcar (nonpowered) V06.10-
three wheeled motor vehicle V02.10-
truck V04.10-
van V03.10-
Injury due to cell phone use Y93.C2
noncollision – *see* Fall, Slip, etc.
unspecified pedestrian accident V09.3-

P (continued)
Pedestrian conveyance – *see also* specific conveyance (roller skates, baby stroller, sled, etc.) V09.9-
collided with other land transport vehicle – *see* V01-V09 with 5th character 9
flat-bottomed pedestrian conveyance NEC – *see also* Snowboard or Snow-skis V00.388-
collided (with)
fixed or stationary object V00.382-
other vehicle or object V00.388-
other flat-bottomed conveyances V00.388-
fell from (on) (on) (off) flat-bottomed conveyance V00.381-
gliding-type pedestrian conveyance NEC – *see also* Ice skates or Sled V00.288-
collided (with)
fixed or stationary object V00.282-
other vehicle or object V00.288-
other gliding-type conveyances V00.288-
fell (from) (on) (off) gliding-type conveyance V00.281-
rolling-type pedestrian conveyance NEC- *see also* roller skates, skateboard, or scooter V00.188-
collided (with)
fixed or stationary object V00.182-
other vehicle or object V00.188-
other rolling-type conveyance V00.188-
fell (from) (on) (off) rolling-type conveyance V00.181-
unspecified pedestrian conveyance V00.898-
collided (with)
fixed or stationary object V0.892-
other vehicle or conveyance V00.898-
fell (from) (on) (off) conveyance V00.891-
injury due to cell phone use Y93.C2

These codes are for <u>accidental</u> injuries. Do not use if injury is due to military or war operations, legal intervention, or medical treatment/complication.

Land Transport Accidents, Traffic – Pick-up Truck or Van

ACCIDENTS - Transport
Land – TRAFFIC V00-V89

P (continued)
Pick-up truck or van V59.9- *see also* Truck
Includes minibus, minivan, sport utility vehicle
patient was DRIVER
collided (with)
animal V50.5-
being ridden V56.5-
animal-drawn vehicle V56.5-
bus V54.5-
car V53.5-
fixed or stationary object V57.5-
heavy transport vehicle V54.5-
hoverboard V59.69-
military vehicle V59.81-
motorcycle V52.5-
motor vehicle NEC V59.69-
motor vehicle NOS V59.60-
other nonmotor vehicle V56.5-
pedal cycle V51.5-
pedestrian (on foot or using conveyance) V50.5-
pick-up truck (two pick-up trucks or pick-up truck and van collided) V53.5-
railway vehicle (train) V55.5-
Segway V59.69-
sport utility vehicle V53.5-
streetcar V56.5-
three-wheeled vehicle V52.5-
truck V54.5-
van (two vans or van and pick-up truck collided) V53.5-
injury (due to) (while)
airbag W22.1-
boarding or alighting pick-up truck or van - *see* Accident, transport, traffic, pick-up truck or van, Occupant
cell phone use Y93.C2
vehicle fire X01.0-
noncollision accident V58.5-
other specified accident V59.49-
unspecified accident V59.40-

If military vehicle involved, use code for military vehicle, **NOT** type of vehicle. For example, patient was driver of pick-up truck collided with military motorcycle. Use code for driver of pick-up truck collided with military vehicle, not driver collided with motorcycle.

P (continued)
Pick-up truck or van V59.9- *see also* Truck
Includes minibus, sport utility vehicle (continued)
patient was HANGER-ON
collided (with)
animal V50.7-
being ridden V56.7-
animal-drawn vehicle V56.7-
bus V54.7-
car V53.7-
fixed or stationary object V57.7-
heavy transport vehicle V54.7-
hoverboard V59.69-
military vehicle V59.81-
motorcycle V52.7-
motor vehicle NEC V59.69-
motor vehicle NOS V59.60-
other nonmotor vehicle V56.7-
pedal cycle V51.7-
pedestrian (on foot or using conveyance) V50.7-
pick-up truck (2 pick-up trucks or pick-up truck and van collided) V53.7-
railway vehicle (train) V55.7-
Segway V59.69-
sport utility vehicle V53.7-
streetcar V56.7-
three wheeled motor vehicle V52.7-
truck V54.7-
van (two vans or van and pick-up truck collided) V53.7-
injury (due to) (while)
boarding or alighting pick-up truck or van - *see* Accident, transport, traffic, pick-up truck or van, occupant
vehicle fire X01.0-
noncollision accident V58.7-
other specified accident V59.59-
unspecified accident V59.50-

List intent/cause codes before other External Cause codes. Use more than one code if needed to completely explain the circumstances. **Use these codes throughout treatment with applicable 7th character.**

ACCIDENTS - Transport
Land – TRAFFIC V00-V89

P (continued)

Pick-up truck or van (continued) (includes sport utility vehicle)
V59.9- - *see also* Truck
- patient was OCCUPANT
  - collided (with)
    - animal V50.9-
      - being ridden V56.9-
    - animal-drawn vehicle V56.9-
    - bus V54.9-
    - car V53.9-
    - fixed or stationary object V57.9-
    - heavy transport vehicle V54.9-
    - hoverboard V59.6-
    - military vehicle V59.81-
    - motorcycle V52.9-
    - other motor vehicle V59.6--
    - other nonmotor vehicle V56.9-
    - pedal cycle V51.9-
    - pedestrian (on foot or using conveyance) V50.9-
    - pick-up truck (two pick-up trucks or pick-up truck and van collided) V53.9-
    - railway vehicle (train) V55.9-
    - Segway V59.6-
    - sport utility vehicle V53.9-
    - streetcar V56.9-
    - three wheeled motor vehicle V52.9-
    - truck V54.9-
    - van (two vans or van and pick-up truck collided) V53.9-
  - injury (due to) (while)
    - airbag W22.19-
    - boarding or alighting pick-up truck or van (collided with)
      - animal V50.4-
        - being ridden V56.4-
      - animal-drawn vehicle V56.4-
      - bus V54.4-
      - car V53.4-
      - fixed or stationary object V57.4-
      - heavy transport vehicle V54.4-
      - motorcycle V52.4-
      - other motor vehicle V59.4-
      - other nonmotor vehicle V56.4-
      - pedal cycle V51.4-
      - pedestrian (on foot) or using conveyance V50.4-
      - pick-up truck V53.4-
      - railway vehicle (train) V55.4-
      - sport utility vehicle or van V53.4-
      - streetcar V56.4-

P (continued)

Pick-up truck or van (continued) (includes sport utility vehicle)
V59.9 - *see also* Truck
- patient was OCCUPANT (continued)
  - injury (due to) (while) (continued)
    - boarding or alighting (collided with) (cont.)
      - three-wheeled vehicle V52.4-
      - truck V54.4-
      - van V53.4-
    - vehicle fire X01.0-
  - noncollision accident V58.9-
    - while boarding or alighting V58.4-
  - other specified accident V59.49-
  - unspecified accident V59.40-
- patient was PASSENGER
  - collided (with)
    - animal V50.6-
      - being ridden V56.6-
    - animal-drawn vehicle V56.6-
    - bus V54.6-
    - car V53.6-
    - fixed or stationary object V57.6-
    - heavy transport vehicle V54.6-
    - hoverboard V59.5-
    - military vehicle V59.81-
    - motorcycle V52.6-
    - other motor vehicle V59.5-
    - other nonmotor vehicle V56.6-
    - pedal cycle V51.6-
    - pedestrian (on foot or using conveyance) V50.6-
    - pick-up truck (two pick-up trucks or pick-up truck and van collided) V53.6-
    - railway vehicle (train) V55.6-
    - Segway V59.5-
    - sport utility vehicle V53.6-
    - streetcar V56.6-
    - three wheeled motor vehicle V52.6-
    - truck V54.6-
    - van (two vans or van and pick-up truck collided) V53.6-
      - injury (due to) (while)
        - airbag W22.12-
        - boarding or alighting – see Accident, transport, traffic, pick-up truck or van, occupant
        - vehicle fire X01.0-
      - noncollision accident V58.6-
      - other specified accident V59.50-
      - unspecified accident V59.59-

Land Transport Accidents, Traffic – Railway vehicle-Roller skates (in-line)

ACCIDENTS - Transport
Land – TRAFFIC V00-V89

R	R (continued)
Railway vehicle (train) (includes subway and elevated train) V81.9- – *see also* Streetcar	**Roller skates (in-line)** (roller blades) V00.118- – *see also* Roller skates (other than in-line)
patient was OCCUPANT (includes engineer, conductor, other crew, passenger, hanger-on)	collided (with)
collided (with)	bus V04.11-
fixed or stationary object V81.3-	car V03.11-
military vehicle V81.83-	fixed or stationary object V00.112-
motor vehicle V81.1-	heavy transport V04.11-
other object V81.3-	military vehicle V09.21-
rolling stock V81.2-	motorcycle V02.11-
railway vehicle (train) V81.2-	other land transport vehicle – *see* V01- V09 with 5th character 9
injury (due to) (while)	other nonmotor vehicle V06.11-
boarding or alighting V81.4-	other object/person V00.118-
cell phone use Y93.C2	pedal cycle V01.11-
derailment of train	pedestrian (on foot or using conveyance) V00.118-
without collision V81.7-	pick-up truck V03.11-
fall after derailment V81.3-	roller skates (two skaters collided) V06.19-
explosion V81.81-	sport utility vehicle V03.11-
fall V81.5-	three wheeled motor vehicle V02.11-
after derailment V81.3-	truck V04.11-
during derailment V81.7-	van V03.11-
fall *from* train V81.6-	injury (due to)
fall *in* train V81.5-	cell phone use Y93.C2
object falling onto train (earth, rocks, stones, etc.) V81.82-	fall (from) (off) V00.111-
vehicle fire V81.81-	noncollision accident V00.118-
other specified accident V81.89-	other accident V00.118-
unspecified accident V81.9-	unspecified accident V00.118-
rickshaw – *see* Accident, transport, traffic, pedal cycle	
rollerblades – *see* roller skates (in-line)	

These codes are used for <u>accidental</u> injuries. Do not use if injury is due to military or war operations, legal intervention Of medical treatment/complication.

ACCIDENTS - Transport
Land – TRAFFIC V00-V89

R (continued)	S
Roller skates (other than in-line) V00.128- – *see also* Roller skates (in-line)	**Scooter** (nonmotorized) (driver, occupant, or passenger) V00.148- If motorized, *see* Motorcycle or Mobility scooter
collided (with)	collided (with)
bus V04.11-	bus V04.19-
car V03.11-	car V03.19-
fixed or stationary object V00.122-	fixed or stationary object V00.142-
heavy transport V04.11-	heavy transport vehicle V04.19-
military vehicle V09.21-	military vehicle V09.21-
motorcycle V02.11-	motorcycle V02.19-
other land transport vehicle – *see* V01- V09 with 5th character 9	other land transport vehicle – *see* V01- V09 with 5th character 9
other nonmotor vehicle V06.11-	other nonmotor vehicle V06.19-
other object/person V00.128-	pedal cycle V01.19-
pedal cycle V01.11-	pedestrian (on foot or using conveyance) V06.19-
pedestrian (on foot or using conveyance) V00.128-	pick-up truck V03.19-
pick-up truck V03.11-	railway vehicle (train) V05.19-
roller skates (2 skaters collided) V00.128-	scooter (nonmotorized) (two scooters collided) V06.19-
sport utility vehicle V03.11-	sport utility vehicle V03.19-
three wheeled motor vehicle V02.11-	streetcar (nonpowered) V06.19-
truck V04.11-	three-wheeled vehicle V02.19-
van V03.11-	truck V04.19-
injury (due to)	van V03.19-
cell phone use Y93.C2	injury (due to)
fall (from) (off) V00.121-	cell phone use Y93.C2
other accident V00.128-	fall (from) (off)
unspecified accident V00.128-	scooter was moving V00.141-
Scooter (motorized) – *see* Accident, transport, traffic, mobility scooter or motorcycle. If not motorized, *see* Scooter, nonmotorized	scooter was not moving W05.1-
	other accident V00.148-
	unspecified accident V00.148-

List intent/cause codes before other External Cause codes. Use more than one code if needed to completely explain the circumstances. **Use these codes throughout treatment with applicable 7th character.**

Land Transport Accidents, Traffic – Segway-Skis

ACCIDENTS - Transport
Land – TRAFFIC V00-V89

S (continued)
Segway V00.848
collided (with)
animal (being ridden) V06.138
animal drawn vehicle V06.138
bus V04.138
car V03.138
fixed or stationary object V00.842
heavy transport vehicle V04.138
hoverboard V06.138
motorcycle V02.138
other motor vehicle V06.138
other nonmotor vehicle V06.138
pedal cycle V01.138
pedestrian (on foot or using conveyance) V06.138
pick-up truck V03.138
railway vehicle (train) V05.138
Segway (two Segways collided) V06.138-
sport utility vehicle V03.138
streetcar (nonpowered) V06.138
three-wheeled vehicle V02.138
truck V04.19-
van V03.138
injury due to cell phone use Y93.C2
fell (from) (off) V00.848
Skateboard V00.138-
collided (with)
animal being ridden V06.12-
animal-drawn vehicle V06.12-
bus V04.12-
car V03.12-
fixed or stationary object V00.132-
heavy transport vehicle V04.12-
military vehicle V09.21-
motorcycle V02.12-
other land transport vehicle – see V01-V09
other nonmotor vehicle V06.12-
pedal cycle V01.12-
pedestrian (on foot or using conveyance) V00.138-
pick-up truck V03.12-
railway vehicle (train) V05.12-

S (continued)
Skateboard V00.138- (continued)
collided (with) (continued)
skateboard (2 skateboards collided) V00.138-
sport utility vehicle V03.12-
three-wheeled vehicle V02.12-
truck V04.12-
van V03.12-
injury (due to)
cell phone use Y93.C2
fall (from) (off) V00.131-
other and unspecified accident V00.138-
Ski lift (any accident) V98.3-
Skis (snow) (for water skis, see Accident, watercraft, water skis) V00.328-
collided (with)
animal being ridden V06.19-
animal-drawn vehicle V06.19-
bus V04.19-
car V03.19-
fixed or stationary object V00.322-
heavy transport vehicle V04.19-
military vehicle V09.21-
motorcycle V02.19-
other land transport vehicle – see V01-V08
other nonmotor vehicle V06.19-
pedal cycle V01.19-
pick-up truck V03.19-
skis (two skiers collided) V00.328-
sport utility vehicle V03.19-
three wheeled vehicle V02.19-
truck V04.19-
van V03.19-
injury (due to)
cell phone use Y93.C2
fall (from) (off) V00.321-
other and unspecified accident V00.328-

If military vehicle involved, use code for military vehicle, **NOT** type of vehicle. For example, patient on skateboard collided military motorcycle. Use code for skateboarder collided with military vehicle, not skateboarder collided with motorcycle.

ACCIDENTS - Transport
Land – TRAFFIC V00-V89

S (continued)
Sled V00.228-
collided (with)
animal being ridden V06.19-
animal-drawn vehicle V06.19-
bus V04.19-
car V03.19-
fixed or stationary object V00.222-
heavy transport vehicle V04.19-
military vehicle V09.21-
motorcycle V02.19-
other land transport vehicle – *see* V01- V09 with 5th character 9
pedal cycle V01.19-
pedestrian (on foot/using conveyance) V00.228-
pick-up truck V03.19-
railway vehicle (train) V05.19-
skis (two skiers collided) V00.228-
sport utility vehicle V03.19-
three wheeled vehicle V02.19-
truck V04.19-
van V03.19-
injury (due to)
cell phone use Y93.C2
fall (off) V00.221-
other and unspecified accident V00.228-
Snowboard V00.318-
collided (with)
animal being ridden V06.19-
animal-drawn vehicle V06.19-
bus V04.19-
car V03.19-
fixed or stationary object V00.312-
heavy transport vehicle V04.19-
military vehicle V09.21-

S (continued)
Snowboard V00.318- (continued)
collided (with) (continued)
motorcycle V02.19-
other land transport vehicle – *see* V01-V09 with 5th character 9
other nonmotor vehicle V06.19-
pedal cycle V01.19-
pedestrian (on foot/using conveyance) V08.318-
pick-up truck V03.19-
railway vehicle (train) V05.19-
sled V00.228-
snowboard (two snowboarders collided) V00.318-
sport utility vehicle V03.19-
three-wheeled vehicle V02.19-
truck V04.19-
van V03.19-
injury (due to)
cell phone use Y93.C2
fall (from) (off) V00.311-
other specified accident V00.318-
unspecified accident V00.318-
Snowmobile V86.32-
injury (due to) (while)
airbag W22.1-
boarding or alighting snowmobile V86.42-
patient was DRIVER V86.02-
patient was HANGER-ON V86.22-
patient was OCCUPANT V86.32-
patient was PASSENGER V86.12-
Sport utility vehicle – *see* Pick-up truck or van
Standing
electric scooter – see Electric scooter
micro-mobility pedestrian conveyance–see hoverboard

These codes are used for <u>accidental</u> injuries. Do not use if injury is due to military or war operations, legal intervention or medical treatment/complication.

Land Transport Accidents, Traffic – Streetcar-Three wheeled vehicle

ACCIDENTS - Transport
Land – TRAFFIC V00-V89

S (continued)
Streetcar (powered) (includes cable car, tram and trolley) (includes conductor, passenger, other crew) V82.8-
collided (with)
animal being ridden V82.8-
animal-drawn vehicle V82.8-
bus V82.1-
car V82.1-
fixed or stationary object V82.3-
heavy transport vehicle V82.1-
military vehicle V82.8-
motorcycle V82.1-
other land transport vehicle – *see* V01-V09
other nonmotor vehicle V82.8-
other object V82.3-
railway vehicle V82.8-
rolling stock V82.2-
Segway V82.1-
streetcar (two streetcars collided) V82.8-
three-wheeled vehicle V82.1-
truck V82.1-
van V82.1-
injury (due to) (while)
boarding or alighting streetcar V82.4-
cell phone use Y93.C2
derailment of streetcar
without collision V82.7-
fall after derailment V82.1-
following collision V82.1-
fall V82.5-
with derailment V82.1-
fall *from* streetcar V82.6-
fall *in* streetcar V82.5-
following collision V82.1-
injury (due to) (while)
cell phone use Y93.C2
vehicle fire X01.0-
other specified accident V82.8-
unspecified accident V82.9-

T
Three wheeled vehicle (motorized) – If vehicle not motorized, *see* pedal cycle V39.9-
patient was DRIVER
collided (with)
animal V30.5-
being ridden V36.5-
animal-drawn vehicle V36.5-
bus V34.5-
car V33.5-
fixed or stationary object V37.5-
heavy transport vehicle V34.5-
hoverboard V39.49-
military vehicle V39.81-
motorcycle V32.5-
motor vehicle NEC V39.49-
motor vehicle NOS V39.40-
other nonmotor vehicle V36.5-
pedal cycle V31.5-
pedestrian (on foot/using conveyance) V30.5-
pick-up truck V33.5-
railway vehicle (train) V35.5-
Segway V39.49-
sport utility vehicle V33.5-
streetcar V36.5-
three-wheeled motor vehicle (2 three-wheeled vehicles collided) V32.5-
truck V34.5-
van V33.5-
injury (due to) (while)
airbag W22.11-
boarding or alighting vehicle – see Accident, transport, traffic, three-wheeled vehicle, occupant
cell phone use Y93.C2
vehicle fire X01.0-
noncollision accident V38.5-
other specified accident V39.89-
unspecified accident V39.9-

List intent/cause codes before other External Cause codes. Use more than one code if needed to completely explain the circumstances. **Use these codes throughout treatment with applicable 7th character.**

ACCIDENTS - Transport
Land – Traffic V00-V89

T (continued)

Three wheeled vehicle (motorized) – If vehicle not motorized, *see* pedal cycle V39.9-
- patient was HANGER-ON
  - collided (with)
    - animal V30.7-
      - being ridden V36.7-
    - animal-drawn vehicle V36.7-
    - bus V34.7-
    - car V33.7-
    - fixed or stationary object V37.7-
    - heavy transport vehicle V34.7-
    - hoverboard V39.49-
    - military vehicle V39.81-
    - motorcycle V32.7-
    - motor vehicle NEC V39.49-
    - motor vehicle NOS V39.40-
    - nonmotor vehicle NEC V36.7-
    - pedal cycle V31.7-
    - pedestrian (on foot/using conveyance) V30.7-
    - pick-up truck V33.7-
    - railway vehicle (train) V35.7-
    - Segway V39.49-
    - sport utility vehicle V33.7-
    - streetcar V36.7-
    - three-wheeled motor vehicle (2 three-wheeled vehicles collided) V32.7-
    - truck V34.7-
    - van V33.7-
  - injury (due to) (while)
    - boarding or alighting vehicle – see Accident, transport, traffic, three-wheeled vehicle, occupant wheeled vehicle, occupant
    - cell phone use Y93.C2
    - vehicle fire X01.0-
  - noncollision accident V38.7-
  - other specified accident V38.89-
  - unspecified accident V39.9-
- patient was OCCUPANT
  - collided (with)
    - animal V30.9-
      - being ridden V36.9-
    - animal-drawn vehicle V36.9-
    - bus V34.9-
    - car V33.9-
    - fixed or stationary object V37.9-
    - heavy transport vehicle V34.9-
    - hoverboard V39.6-

T (continued)

Three wheeled vehicle (motorized) – If vehicle not motorized, *see* pedal cycle V39.9- (continued)
- patient was OCCUPANT (continued)
  - collided (with) (continued)
    - military vehicle V39.81-
    - motorcycle V32.9-
    - other motor vehicle V39.6-
    - other nonmotor vehicle V36.60-
    - pedal cycle V31.9-
    - pedestrian (on foot/using conveyance) V30.9-
    - pick-up truck V33.9-
    - railway vehicle (train) V35.9-
    - Segway V39.6-
    - sport utility vehicle V33.9-
    - streetcar V36.9-
    - three-wheeled motor vehicle (2 three-wheeled vehicles collided) V32.9-
    - truck V34.9-
    - van V33.9-
  - injury (due to) (while)
    - airbag W22.1-
    - boarding or alighting vehicle (collided with)
      - animal V30.4-
        - being ridden V36.4-
      - animal-drawn vehicle V36.4-
      - bus V34.4-
      - car V33.4-
      - fixed or stationary object V37.4-
      - heavy transport vehicle V34.4-
      - motorcycle V32.4-
      - other nonmotor vehicle V36.4-
      - pedal cycle V31.4-
      - pedestrian (on foot/using conveyance)- V30.4-
      - pick-up truck V33.4-
      - railway vehicle (train) V35.4-
      - sport utility vehicle V33.4-
      - streetcar V36.4-
      - three wheeled vehicle V32.4-
      - truck V34.4-
      - van V33.4-
    - vehicle fire X01.0-
  - noncollision accident V38.9-
    - while boarding or alighting vehicle V38.4-
  - other specified accident V39.89-
  - unspecified accident V39.9-

Land Transport Accidents, Traffic – Three wheeled vehicle-Truck

ACCIDENTS - Transport
Land – TRAFFIC V00-V89

T (continued)
Three wheeled vehicle (motorized) – If vehicle not motorized, see pedal cycle V39.9- (continued)
patient was PASSENGER
collided (with)
animal V30.6-
being ridden V36.6-
animal-drawn vehicle V36.6-
bus V34.6-
car V33.6-
fixed or stationary object V37.6-
heavy transport vehicle V34.6-
hoverboard V39.5-
military vehicle V39.81-
motorcycle V32.6-
other motor vehicle V39.5-
other nonmotor vehicle V36.6-
pedal cycle V31.6-
pedestrian (on foot/using conveyance) V30.6-
pick-up truck V33.6-
railway vehicle (train) V35.6-
Segway V39.5-
streetcar V36.6-
three-wheeled motor vehicle (2 three-wheeled vehicles collided) V32.6-
truck V34.6-
van V33.6-
injury (due to) (while)
airbag W22.12-
boarding or alighting vehicle – see Accident, transport, traffic, three-wheeled vehicle, occupant
vehicle fire X01.0-
noncollision accident V38.6-
other specified accident V39.89-
unspecified accident V39.9-
Tractor (and trailer) – see Accident, transport, traffic, agricultural vehicle
Train – see Accident, transport, traffic, railway vehicle
Tram – see Accident, transport, traffic, streetcar
Tricycle - see Accident, transport, traffic, pedal cycle
motorized - see Accident, transport, traffic, three-wheeled vehicle
Trolley —see Accident, transport, traffic, streetcar

T (continued)
Truck (18-wheeler, armored or paneled truck, heavy transport vehicle) – see also Pick-up truck or van V69.9-
patient was DRIVER
collided (with)
animal V60.5-
being ridden V66.5-
animal-drawn vehicle V66.5-
bus V64.5-
car V63.5-
fixed or stationary object V67.5-
heavy transport vehicle V64.5-
hoverboard V69.49-
military vehicle V69.81-
motorcycle V62.5-
motor vehicle NEC V69.49-
motor vehicle NOS V69.40-
other nonmotor vehicle V66.5-
pedal cycle V61.5-
pedestrian (on foot or using conveyance) V60.5-
pick-up truck V63.5-
railway vehicle (train) V65.5-
Segway V69.49-
sport utility vehicle V63.5-
streetcar V66.5-
three-wheeled motor vehicle V62.5-
truck (two trucks collided) V64.5-
van V63.5-
injury (due to) (while)
airbag W22.11-
boarding or alighting truck - see Accident, transport, truck, occupant
cell phone use Y93.C2
vehicle fire X01.0-
noncollision accident V68.5-
other specified accidents NEC V69.49-
unspecified accident V69.40-

If military vehicle involved, use code for military vehicle **NOT** type of vehicle. For example, patient was truck driver who collided with military motorcycle. Use code for truck driver collided with military vehicle, not truck driver collided with motorcycle.

ACCIDENTS - Transport
Land – TRAFFIC V00-V89

T (continued)

Truck (18-wheeler, armored or paneled truck, heavy transport vehicle) V69.9- *see also* Pick-up truck or van
- patient was HANGER-ON
  - collided (with)
    - animal V60.7-
      - being ridden V66.7-
    - animal-drawn vehicle V66.7-
    - bus V64.7-
    - car V63.7-
    - fixed or stationary object V67.7-
    - heavy transport vehicle V64.7-
    - hoverboard V69.69-
    - military vehicle V69.81-
    - motorcycle V62.7-
    - motor vehicle NEC V69.69-
    - motor vehicle NOS V64.60-
    - other nonmotor vehicle V66.7-
    - pedal cycle V61.7-
    - pedestrian (on foot or using conveyance) V60.7-
    - pick-up truck V63.7-
    - railway vehicle (train) V65.7-
    - Segway V69.69-
    - sport utility vehicle V63.7-
    - streetcar V66.7-
    - three-wheeled motor vehicle V62.7-
    - truck (two trucks collided) V64.7-
    - van V63.7-
  - injury (due to) (while)
    - boarding or alighting truck - see Accident, transport, traffic, truck, occupant
    - vehicle fire X01.0-
  - noncollision accident V68.7-
  - other specified accident V69.69-
  - unspecified accident V69.60
- patient was OCCUPANT
  - collided (with)
    - animal V60.9-
      - being ridden V66.9-
    - animal-drawn vehicle V66.9-
    - bus V64.9-
    - car V63.9-
    - fixed or stationary object V67.9-
    - heavy transport vehicle V64.9-
    - hoverboard V69.6-

T (continued)

Truck (18-wheeler, armored or paneled truck, heavy transport vehicle) V69.9- see also Pick-up truck or van (continued)
- patient was OCCUPANT (continued)
  - collided (with) (continued)
    - military vehicle V69.81-
    - motorcycle V62.9-
    - other motor vehicle V69.6-
    - other nonmotor vehicle V66.9-
    - pedal cycle V61.9-
    - pedestrian (on foot/using conveyance) V60.9-
    - pick-up truck V63.9-
    - railway vehicle (train) V65.9-
    - Segway V69.6-
    - sport utility vehicle V63.9-
    - streetcar V66.9-
    - three-wheeled motor vehicle V62.9-
    - truck (two trucks collided) V64.9-
    - van V63.9-
  - injury (due to) (while)
    - airbag W22.1-
    - boarding or alighting (collided with)
      - animal V60.4-
        - being ridden V66.4-
      - animal-drawn vehicle V66.4-
      - bus V64.4-
      - car V63.4-
      - fixed or stationary object V67.4-
      - heavy transport vehicle V64.4-
      - motorcycle V62.4-
      - other nonmotor vehicle V66.4-
      - pedal cycle V61.4-
      - pedestrian (on foot/using conveyance) V60.4-
      - pick-up truck V63.4-
      - railway vehicle (train) V65.4-
      - sports utility vehicle
      - streetcar V66.4-
      - three-wheeled vehicle V62.4-
      - truck V64.4-
      - van V63.4-
    - vehicle fire X01.0-
  - noncollision accident V68.9-
    - while board or alighting truck V68.4-
  - other specified accident V69.69-
  - unspecified accident V69.60-

These codes are used for <u>accidental</u> injuries. Do not use if injury is due to military or war operations, legal intervention or medical treatment/complication.

Land Transport Accidents, Traffic – Truck-Unknown vehicle

ACCIDENTS - Transport
Land – TRAFFIC V00-V89

T (continued)	U
Truck (18-wheeler, armored or paneled truck) – V69.9- see also Pick-up truck or van (continued)	**Unknown vehicle** (vehicles involved in accident known but not which vehicle was patient's) V89.9-
patient was PASSENGER	collision involved
collided (with)	bus and
animal V60.6-	car V87.3-
being ridden V66.6-	heavy transport vehicle V87.5-
animal-drawn vehicle V66.6-	motorcycle V87.1-
bus V64.6-	three-wheeled vehicle V87.1-
car V63.6-	car and
fixed or stationary object V67.6-	bus V87.3-
heavy transport vehicle V64.6-	heavy transport vehicle V87.4-
hoverboard V69.5-	motorcycle V87.0-
military vehicle V69.81-	pick-up truck V87.2-
motorcycle V62.6-	railway vehicle (train) V87.6-
other motor vehicle V69.5-	three-wheeled vehicle V87.0-
other nonmotor vehicle V66.1-	van V87.2-
pedal cycle V61.6-	heavy transport vehicle and
pedestrian (on foot/using conveyance) V60.6-	bus V87.5-
pick-up truck V63.6-	car V87.4-
railway vehicle (train) V65.6-	motorcycle and
Segway V69.5-	car V87.0-
sport utility vehicle V63.6-	other motor vehicle and
streetcar V66.6-	motorcycle V87.1-
three-wheeled motor vehicle V62.6-	three-wheeled vehicle V87.1-
truck (two trucks collided) V64.6-	pick-up truck and
van V63.6-	car V87.2-
injury (due to) (while)	railway vehicle (train) and
airbag W22.12-	car V87.6-
boarding or alighting truck–see Accident, transport, traffic, truck, occupant	three-wheeled vehicle and
	bus V87.1-
vehicle fire X01.0-	car V87.0-
noncollision accident V68.6-	van and
other specified accident V69.59-	bus V87.2-
unspecified accident V69.50-	car V87.2-
Two-wheeled vehicle (motorized) – see Accident, transport, traffic, motorcycle. If not motorized, see Pedal cycle	noncollision accident involving
	motor vehicle NEC V87.8-
	nonmotor vehicle NOS V87.9-
	other accident involving
	other motor vehicle V87.7-
	pedal cycle – see V10-V19
	pedestrian – see V01-V09

List intent/cause codes before other External Cause codes. Use more than one code if needed to completely explain The circumstances. Use these codes throughout treatment with applicable 7th character.

ACCIDENTS - Transport
Land – TRAFFIC V00-V89

V
Van – *see* Pick-up truck

W
Walking – *see* Pedestrian (on foot)
Wheelchair (powered) V00.818-
collided (with)
bus V04.19-
car V03.19-
fixed or stationary object V00.812-
heavy transport vehicle V04.19-
military vehicle V09.21-
motorcycle V02.19-
other land transport vehicle – *see* V01-V09
other nonmotor vehicle V06.19-
pedestrian (on foot/using pedestrian conveyance) V00.09-
pick-up truck V03.19-
railway vehicle (train) V05.19-
sport utility vehicle V03.19-
three-wheeled motor vehicle V02.19-
truck V04.19-
van V03.19-
wheelchair (two wheelchairs collided) V00.818-
injury (due to) (while)
boarding or alighting wheelchair V00.818-
cell phone use Y93.C2
fall (from) (out)
wheelchair was moving V00.811-
wheelchair was not moving W05.0-
noncollision accident V00.818-
other specified accident V00.818-
unspecified accident V00.818-
Wheeled shoes – *see* Heelies

If military vehicle involved, use code for military vehicle, **NOT** type of vehicle. For example, wheelchair rider collided with military motorcycle. Use code for wheelchair collided with military vehicle, not wheelchair collided with motorcycle.

END OF INJURY, ACCIDENT, TRANSPORT, TRAFFIC

Land Transport Accidents, Unspecified – Baby stroller-Pedestrian

ACCIDENTS - Transport
Land – UNSPECIFIED Traffic/Nontraffic V00-V89

B	M
Baby stroller V00.828-	**Mobility scooter** (driver, passenger, or occupant) (motorized) V00.838-
collided (with)	collided (with)
bus V04.99-	bus V04.99-
car V03.99-	car V03.99-
heavy transport vehicle V04.99-	heavy transport vehicle V04.99-
motorcycle V02.99-	motorcycle V02.99-
other land transport vehicle – *see* V01-V09	other land transport vehicle – *see* V01-V09
other nonmotor vehicle V06.99-	other nonmotor vehicle V06.99-
pedal cycle V01.99-	pedal cycle V01.99-
pick-up truck V03.99-	pick-up truck V03.99-
railway vehicle (train) V05.99-	railway vehicle (train) V05.99-
sport utility vehicle V03.99-	sport utility vehicle V03.99-
three-wheeled motor vehicle V02.99-	three-wheeled motor vehicle V02.99-
van V03.99-	van V03.99-
other baby stroller accident (injury due to)	other mobility scooter accident (injury due to)
cell phone use Y93.C2	airbag W22.1-
other baby stroller accident V00.828-	cell phone use Y93.C2
I	fall (from) (off) V00.831-
Ice skates V00.218--	vehicle fire X01.0-
collided (with)	other mobility scooter accident V00.838-
bus V04.99-	**P**
car V03.99-	**Pedestrian (on foot)** V09.9-
heavy transport vehicle V04.99-	collided (with)
motorcycle V02.99-	bus V04.90-
other land transport vehicle – *see* V01-V09	car V03.90-
other nonmotor vehicle V06.99-	heavy transport vehicle V04.90-
pedal cycle V01.99-	motorcycle V02.90-
pick-up truck V03.99-	other land transport vehicle – *see* V01-V09
railway vehicle (train) V05.99-	other nonmotor vehicle V06.90-
sport utility vehicle V03.99-	pedal cycle V01.90-
three-wheeled motor vehicle V02.99-	pick-up truck V03.90-
van V03.99-	railway vehicle (train) V05.90-
other ice skating accident (injury due to)	sport utility vehicle V03.90-
cell phone use Y93.C2	three-wheeled motor vehicle V02.90-
other ice skating accident V00.218-	van V03.90-
	other pedestrian accident (injury due to)
	cell phone use Y93.C2
	other pedestrian accident V09.9-

Note: Assume accident was in traffic if not listed here.

These codes are listed for <u>accidental</u> injuries. Do not use
If injury is due to military or war operations, legal
Intervention or medical treatment/complication.

ACCIDENTS - Transport
Land – UNSPECIFIED Traffic/Nontraffic V00-V89

R		S (continued)	
Roller-skates (roller blades) V00.1-		**Skateboard** V00.138-	
	collided (with)		collided (with)
	bus V04.91-		bus V04.92-
	car V03.91-		car V03.92-
	heavy transport vehicle V04.91-		heavy transport vehicle V04.92-
	motorcycle V02.91-		motorcycle V02.92-
	other land transport vehicle – see V01-V09		other land transport vehicle – see V01-V09
	other nonmotor vehicle V06.91-		other nonmotor vehicle V06.92-
	pedal cycle V01.91-		pedal cycle V01.92-
	pick-up truck V03.91-		pick-up truck V03.92-
	railway vehicle (train) V05.91-		railway vehicle (train) V05.92-
	sport utility vehicle V03.91-		sport utility vehicle V03.92-
	three-wheeled motor vehicle V02.91-		three-wheeled motor vehicle V02.92-
	van V03.91-		van V03.92-
other roller skate accident (injury due to)		other skateboard accident (injury due to)	
	cell phone use Y93.C2		cell phone use Y93.C2
	in-line skates (roller blades) V00.118-		other skateboarding accident V00.138-
	non-in-line skates V00.128-	**Skis (snow)** V00.388-	
S			collided (with)
Scooter (nonmotorized) V00.838- If motorized, see Motorcycle or Mobility Scooter			bus V04.99-
			car V03.99-
	collided (with)		heavy transport vehicle V04.99-
	bus V04.99-		motorcycle V02.99-
	car V03.99-		other land transport vehicle – see V01-V09 with 5th character 9
	heavy transport vehicle V04.99-		
	motorcycle V02.99-		pedal cycle V01.99-
	other land transport vehicle – see V01-V09		pick-up truck V03.99-
	other nonmotor vehicle V06.99-		railway vehicle (train) V05.99-
	pedal cycle V01.99-		sport utility vehicle V03.99-
	pick-up truck V03.99-		three-wheeled motor vehicle V02.99-
	railway vehicle (train) V05.99-		van V03.99-
	sport utility vehicle V03.99-	other scooter accident (injury due to)	
	three-wheeled motor vehicle V02.99-		cell phone use Y93.C2
	van V03.99-		Other ski accident Y00.388-
other scooter accident (injury due to)			
	cell phone use Y93.C2		
	other scooter accident V00.838-		

List intent/cause codes before other External Cause codes. Use more than one code if needed to completely explain The circumstances. **Use these codes throughout treatment with applicable 7th character.**

Land Transport Accidents, Unspecified – Sled-Wheelchair

ACCIDENTS - Transport
Land – UNSPECIFIED Traffic/Nontraffic V00-V89

S (continued)	
Sled V00.228-	
	collided (with)
	bus V04.99-
	car V03.99-
	heavy transport vehicle V04.99-
	motorcycle V02.99-
	other land transport vehicle – *see* V01-V09 other nonmotor vehicle V06.99-
	pedal cycle V01.99-
	pick-up truck V03.99-
	railway vehicle (train) V05.99-
	sport utility vehicle V03.99-
	three-wheeled motor vehicle V02.99-
	van V03.99-
	other sledding accident (injury due to)
	cell phone use Y93.C2
	other sledding accident V00.228-
Snowboard V00.318-	
	collided (with)
	bus V04.99-
	car V03.99-
	heavy transport vehicle V04.99-
	motorcycle V02.99-
	other land transport vehicle – *see* V01-V09 with 5th character 9
	other nonmotor vehicle V06.99-
	pick-up truck V03.99
	railway vehicle (train) V05.99-
	sport utility vehicle V03.99-
	three-wheeled motor vehicle V02.99-
	van V03.99-
	other snowboard accident (injury due to)
	cell phone use Y93.C2
	other snowboarding accident V00.318-

W	
Wheelchair (powered) V00.818-	
	collided (with)
	bus V04.99-
	car V03.99-
	heavy transport vehicle V04.99-
	motorcycle V02.99-
	other land transport vehicle – *see* V01-
	other nonmotor vehicle V06.99-V09 with 5th character 9
	pick-up truck V03.99-
	railway vehicle (train) V05.99-
	sport utility vehicle V03.99-
	three-wheeled motor vehicle V02.99-
	van V03.99-
	other wheelchair accident (injury due to)
	cell phone use Y93.C2
	other wheelchair accident V00.818-

Note: Assume accident was in traffic if not listed here.

If military vehicle involved, use code for military vehicle **NOT** Type of vehicle. For example, wheelchair rider collided with military motorcycle. Use code for wheelchair collided with military vehicle, not wheelchair collided with motorcycle.

END OF INJURY, ACCIDENTAL INTENT, TRANSPORT, UNSPECIFIED AS NONTRAFFIC OR TRAFFIC

Accidents, Watercraft – Air mattress-Fishing boat

ACCIDENTS - Transport
Watercraft V90-V94

A	
Air mattress – *see* Inflatable watercraft	

C	
Canoe (includes kayak) V91.85-	
patient burned (due to)	
	without accident to canoe/kayak V93.19-
	canoe/kayak on fire V91.05-
	other burn (not involving fire onboard) V93.19-
patient drowned or submerged (due to) (following)	
	fall or jump (from canoe/kayak) (into water)
	burning canoe/kayak V90.25-
	crushed canoe/kayak V90.35-
	hitting object or bottom of body of water V94.0-
	other accident resulting in drowning or submersion V90.85-
	overturned canoe/kayak V90.05-
	sinking canoe/kayak V90.15-
	thrown overboard by motion of watercraft V92.15-
	washed overboard V92.25-
patient injured (due to accident onboard)	
	collision (with other watercraft or object (resulting in) (without drowning or submersion)
		fall V91.25-
		patient crushed between canoe and other watercraft or object V91.15-
			fall V93.35-
			heat exposure V93.29-
	hit or struck (by) (patient in watercraft)
		falling object V93.48-
		nonpowered watercraft V94.21-
		powered watercraft V94.22-
	patient in water (after fall from craft) hit by
		powered watercraft V94.11-
		unpowered watercraft V94.12-
Cruise ship – *see* Passenger ship	

F	
Ferry boat – *see* Passenger ship	
Fishing boat (powered) V91.82-	
patient burned (due to)	
	without accident to fishing boat V93.02-
	fishing boat on fire V91.02-
		localized (small) fire on fishing boat V93.02-
		other burn (not due to fire onboard) V93.12-
patient drowned or submerged (due to) (following)	
	fall or jump (from) (into water)
		burning fishing boat V90.22-
		crushed fishing boat V90.32-
		hitting object or bottom of body of water V94.0-
		other fall off (out of) fishing boat V92.02-
	other accident resulting in drowning or submersion V90.82-
		overturned fishing boat V90.02-
		sinking fishing boat V90.12-
		thrown overboard by motion of boat V92.12-
		washed overboard V92.22-
patient injured (due to accident onboard ferry boat)	
	explosion V93.52-
	heat exposure V93.22-
	hit or struck by falling object V91.32-
	machinery onboard causing injury V93.62-
	patient crushed between ferry and other watercraft or object V91.12-
patient in water (after fall from boat) hit by	
	powered watercraft V94.11-
	unpowered watercraft V94.12-
patient on watercraft being pulled behind fishing boat	
	patient on recreational watercraft V94.31-
	patient on nonrecreational watercraft (dingy, life-raft) V94.32-

These codes are used for <u>accidental</u> injuries. Do not use if injury is due to military or war operations, legal Intervention or medical treatment/complications.

Accidents, Watercraft – Inflatable-Liner

ACCIDENTS - Transport
Watercraft V90-V94

I
Inflatable watercraft (raft, air mattress, tube) V91.86-
patient burned (due to)
without accident to watercraft V93.19-
watercraft on fire V91.06-
other burn (not involving fire onboard) V93.19-
patient drowned or submerged (due to) (following)
fall or jump (from watercraft) (into water)
burning watercraft V90.26-
crushed watercraft V90.36-
hitting object or bottom of body of water V94.0-
other accident resulting in drowning or submersion V90.86-
overturned watercraft V90.06-
sinking watercraft V90.16-
thrown overboard by motion of watercraft V92.16-
washed overboard V92.26-
patient injured (due to accident onboard watercraft)
collision (with another watercraft or object) (resulting in) (without drowning or submersion)
fall V91.26-
patient crushed between watercraft other watercraft or object V91.16-
fall V93.36-
heat exposure V93.29-
hit or struck by (patient on watercraft)
falling object V93.48-
nonpowered watercraft V94.21-
powered watercraft V94.22-
patient in water (after fall from watercraft) hit by
powered watercraft V94.11-
unpowered watercraft V94.12-
patient being pulled behind other watercraft
patient on recreational watercraft V94.31-
patient on nonrecreational watercraft (dingy, life-raft) V94.32-
Inner tube – see Inflatable watercraft

J
Jet skis V81.83-
patient burned (due to)
without accident to jet skis V93.03-
jet skis on fire V91.03-
localized (small) fire on jet skis V93.03-
other burn (not related to fire onboard) V93.13-
patient drowned or submerged (due to) (following)
fall or jump (from)
burning jet skis V90.23-
crushed jet skis V90.33-
hitting object or bottom of body of water V94.0-
other fall off jet skis V92.03-
other accidents resulting in drowning or submersion
overturned jet ski V90.03-
sinking jet ski V90.13-
Washed overboard V92.23-
patient injured (due to accident on jet skis)
explosion V93.53-
fall V91.23-
heat exposure V93.23-
hit or struck by falling object V91.33-
machinery onboard causing injury V93.63-
patient crushed between jet skis and other watercraft or object V91.13-
patient in water (after fall from skis) hit by
powered watercraft V94.11-
unpowered watercraft V94.12-
patient on watercraft being pulled behind jet skis
patient on recreational watercraft V94.31-
patient on nonrecreational watercraft (dingy,
K
Kayak – see Canoe
L
Life-raft – see Inflatable watercraft
Liner – see Passenger ship

List intent/cause codes before other External Cause codes. Use more than one code if needed to completely explain the circumstances. **Use these codes throughout treatment with applicable 7th character.**

Accidents, Watercraft – Merchant ship-Raft

ACCIDENTS - Transport
Watercraft V90-V94

M
Merchant ship V91.80-
patient burned (due to)
without accident to ship V93.00-
localized (small) fire on ship V93.00-
other burn (not related to fire onboard) V93.10-
ship on fire V91.00-
patient drowned or submerged (due to) (following)
fall or jump (from ship) (into water)
burning ship V90.20-
crushed ship V90.30-
hitting head on object or bottom of body of water V94.0-
other fall off (out of) ship V92.00-
other accident resulting in drowning or submersion V90.80-
overturned ship V90.00-
sinking ship V90.10-
thrown overboard by motion of ship V92.10-
washed overboard V92.20-
patient injured (due to)
explosion V93.50-
heat exposure V93.20-
hit or struck by falling object V93.40-
machinery onboard causing injury V93.60-
patient crushed between ship and other watercraft or object V91.10-
patient in water (after fall from ship) hit by
powered watercraft V94.11-
unpowered watercraft V94.12-
patient on watercraft being pulled behind merchant Ship
patient on recreational watercraft V94.31-
patient on nonrecreational watercraft (dingy, life-raft) V94.32-
Military watercraft V94.818-
patient in civilian watercraft injured in accident with military watercraft V94.810-
patient (civilian) in water injured in accident with military watercraft V94.811-
patient on recreational watercraft V94.31-
patient on nonrecreational watercraft (dingy, life-raft) V94.32-
other accident involving military watercraft V94.818

O
Ocean liner – see Passenger ship

P
Passenger ship (includes ferry boat, ocean liner, cruise ship) V91.81-
patient burned (due to)
without accident to ship V93.01-
ship on fire V91.01-
localized (small) fire on ship V93.01-
other burn (not due to fire onboard) V93.11-
patient drowned or submerged (due to) (following)
fall or jump (from)
burning ship V90.21-
crushed ship V90.31-
hitting object or bottom of body of water V94.0-
other fall off (out of) ship V92.01-
other accident resulting in drowning or submersion V90.81-
overturned ship V90.01-
sinking ship V90.11-
thrown overboard by motion of ship V92.11-
washed overboard V92.21-
patient injured (due to)
explosion V93.51-
heat exposure V93.21-
hit or struck by falling object V91.31-
machinery onboard causing injury V93.61-
patient crushed between ship and other watercraft or object V91.11-
patient in water (after fall from ship) hit by
powered watercraft V94.11-
unpowered watercraft V94.12-
patient on craft being pulled behind ship
patient on recreational watercraft V94.31
patient on nonrecreational watercraft (dingy, life-raft) V94.32-

R
Raft (inflatable) - see Inflatable watercraft

These codes are for <u>accidental</u> injuries. Do not use if injury is due to military or war operations, legal intervention Or medical treatment/complication.

Accidents, Watercraft – Sailboat-Tube

ACCIDENTS - Transport
Watercraft V90-V94

S
Sailboat V91.84-
patient burned (due to)
without accident to sailboat V93.14-
sailboat on fire V93.04-
other burn V91.14-
patient drowned or submerged (due to) (following)
fall or jump (from sailboat) (into water)
burning sailboat V90.24-
crushed sailboat V90.34-
hitting object or bottom of body of water V94.0-
other accident resulting in drowning or submersion V90.84-
overturned sailboat V90.04-
sinking sailboat V90.14-
thrown overboard by motion of sailboat V92.14-
washed overboard V92.24-
patient injured (due to accident onboard sailboat)
collision (with other watercraft of object) (resulting in) (without drowning or submersion)
fall V91.24-
patient crushed between watercraft or object V91.14-
fall V93.34-
heat exposure V93.24-
hit or struck by (patient on sailboat)
falling object V93.44-
nonpowered watercraft V94.24-
powered watercraft V94.22-
patient in water (after fall from sailboat)
powered watercraft V94.11-
unpowered watercraft V94.12-
patient being pulled behind sailboat
patient on recreational watercraft V94.31-
patient on nonrecreational watercraft (dingy, life-raft) V94.32-
Skis- *see* Water skis

S (continued)
Surfboard (includes windsurf boarding) V91.88-
patient burned (due to)
without accident to board V93.19-
surfboard on fire V91.08-
other burn V93.18-
patient drowned or submerged (due to) (following)
fall or jump (from surfboard) (into water)
burning board V90.28-
crushed board V90.38-
hitting object or bottom of body of water V94.0-
other accident resulting in drowning or submersion V90.88-
overturned board V90.08-
sinking board V90.18-
thrown overboard by motion of board V92.19-
washed overboard V92.28-
patient injured (due to accident on board)
collision (with other watercraft of object) (resulting in) (without drowning or submersion)
fall V93.38-
patient crushed between watercraft or object V91.18-
heat exposure V93.29-
hit or struck by (patient on board)
falling object V93.48-
nonpowered watercraft V94.21-
powered watercraft V94.22-
patient in water (after fall from board)
powered watercraft V94.11-
unpowered watercraft V94.12-
Swimmer (hit by)
powered watercraft V94.11-
unpowered watercraft V94.12-
T
Tube (inflatable) (inner) see inflatable craft

List intent/cause codes before External Cause codes. Use more than one code if needed to completely explain the circumstances. **Use these codes throughout treatment with applicable 7th character.**

Accidents, Watercraft – Water skis-Watercraft (powered) NEC

ACCIDENTS - Transport
Watercraft V90-V94

W
Water skis V91.87-
patient burned (due to)
without accident to water skis V93.19-
other burn V93.19-
water skis on fire V93.09-
patient drowned or submerged (due to) (following)
fall or jump (from skis) (into water)
burning skis V90.27-
crushed skis V90.37-
hitting object or bottom of body of water V94.0-
other accident resulting in drowning or submersion V90.87-
overturned skis V90.08-
sinking skis V90.18-
thrown overboard by motion of skis V92.19-
washed overboard V92.27-
patient injured (due to accident on skis)
barefoot water-skier injured V94.4-
collision (with other watercraft or object) (resulting in) (without drowning or submersion)
fall V91.29-
patient crushed between watercraft and object V91.18-
fall V93.38-
heat exposure V93.29-
hit or struck by (patient on skis)
falling object V93.48-
nonpowered watercraft V94.21-
powered watercraft V94.22-
patient in water (after fall from skis) hit by
powered watercraft V94.11-
unpowered watercraft V94.12-

W (continued)
Watercraft (powered) NEC V91.83-
patient burned (due to)
without accident to watercraft V93.13-
localized (small) fire on watercraft V93.03-
other burn (not due to fire onboard) V93.19-
watercraft on fire V91.03-
patient drowned or submerged (due to) (following)
fall or jump (from watercraft) (into water)
burning watercraft V90.23-
crushed watercraft V90.33-
hitting object or bottom of body of water V94.0-
other accident resulting in drowning or submersion V90.83-
overturned watercraft V90.03-
sinking watercraft V90.13-
thrown overboard by motion of watercraft V92.13-
washed overboard V92.23-
patient injured (due to accident on watercraft)
collision (with another watercraft or object) (resulting in) (without drowning or submersion)
fall V91.23-
patient crushed between watercraft or object V91.13-
explosion V93.53-
fall (without collision) V93.33-
heat exposure V93.23-
hit or struck by falling object V91.33-
machinery onboard causing injury V93.63-
patient in water (after fall from watercraft hit by
powered watercraft V94.11-
unpowered watercraft V94.12-
patient being pulled behind watercraft NEC
patient on recreational watercraft V94.31-
patient on nonrecreational watercraft (dingy, life-raft) V94.32-

These codes are used for <u>accidental</u> injuries. Do not use if Injury due to military or war operations, legal intervention or medical treatment/complication.

Accidents, Watercraft – Watercraft (powered) NOS-Watercraft (unpowered) NEC

ACCIDENTS - Transport
Watercraft V90-V94

W (continued)
Watercraft (powered) NOS V91.89-
patient burned (due to)
without accident to watercraft V93.19-
localized (small) fire on watercraft V93.09-
other burn (not due to fire onboard) V93.19-
watercraft on fire V91.09-
patient drowned or submerged (due to) (following)
fall or jump (from watercraft) (into water)
burning watercraft V90.29-
crushed watercraft V90.39-
hitting object or bottom of body of water V94.0-
other accident resulting in drowning or submersion V90.89-
overturned watercraft V90.09-
sinking watercraft V90.19-
thrown overboard by motion of watercraft V92.19-
washed overboard V92.29-
patient injured (due to accident onboard watercraft)
collision (with another watercraft or object) (resulting in) (without drowning or submersion)
fall V91.29-
patient crushed between watercraft or object V91.19-
explosion V93.59-
fall V93.39-
heat exposure V93.29-
hit or struck by object V93.39-
machinery onboard causing injury V93.69-
patient in water (after fall from watercraft) hit by
powered watercraft V94.11-
unpowered watercraft V94.12-
patient on watercraft being pulled behind watercraft NOS
patient on recreational watercraft V94.31-
patient on nonrecreational watercraft (dingy, life-raft) V94.32-

W (continued)
Watercraft (unpowered) NEC V91.88-
patient burned (due to)
without accident to watercraft V93.19-
other burn V93.19-
watercraft on fire V93.09-
patient drowned or submerged (due to) (following)
fall or jump (from watercraft) (into water)
burning watercraft V90.28-
crushed watercraft V90.38-
hitting object or bottom of body of water V94.0-
other accident resulting in drowning or submersion V90.88-
overturned watercraft V90.08-
sinking watercraft V90.18-
thrown overboard by motion of watercraft V92.19-
washed overboard V92.28-
patient injured (due to accident onboard watercraft)
collision (with another watercraft or object (resulting in) (without drowning or submersion)
fall V91.29-
patient crushed between watercraft and object V91.18-
fall V93.38-
heat exposure V93.29-
hit or struck by (patient on/in watercraft)
falling object V93.48-
nonpowered watercraft V94.21-
powered watercraft V94.22-
patient in water (after fall from watercraft) hit by
powered watercraft V94.11-
unpowered watercraft V94.12-
patient being pulled behind watercraft NEC
patient on recreational watercraft V94.31-
patient on nonrecreational watercraft (dingy, life-raft) V94.32-

List intent/cause codes before other External Cause codes. Use more than one code if needed to completely explain the circumstances. **Use these codes throughout treatment with applicable 7th character.**

Accidents, Watercraft – Watercraft (powered) NOS-Windsurfing

ACCIDENTS - Transport
Watercraft V90-V94

W (continued)	W (continued)
Watercraft (unpowered) NOS V91.89-	**Windsurfing** – *see* Surfboard
patient burned (due to)	
without accident to watercraft V93.19-	
other burn V93.19-	
watercraft on fire V93.09-	
patient drowned or submerged (due to) (following)	
fall or jump (from watercraft) (into water)	
burning watercraft V90.29-	
crushed watercraft V90.39-	
hitting head on object or bottom of body of water V94.0-	
other accident resulting in drowning or submersion V90.89-	These codes are used for <u>accidental</u> injuries.
overturned watercraft V90.09-	Do not use if injury due to military or war operations,
sinking watercraft V90.19-	Legal intervention or medical treatment/complication.
thrown overboard by motion of watercraft V92.19-	
washed overboard V92.29-	
patient injured (due to accident on watercraft)	
collision (with other watercraft or object) (resulting in) (without drowning or submersion)	
fall V91.29-	
fall V93.39-	
heat exposure V93.29-	
hit or struck by falling object (patient in watercraft) V93.49-	
patient crushed between watercraft and object V91.19-	
patient in water (after fall from watercraft) hit by	
powered watercraft V94.11-	
unpowered watercraft V94.12-	
patient being pulled behind watercraft NOS	
patient on recreational watercraft V94.31-	
patient on nonrecreational watercraft V94.32-	

END OF INJURY, ACCIDENTAL INTENT, TRANSPORT

Accidents, Other Adverse effects-Bumping into

CATEGORY – INTENT/CAUSE - ACCIDENTS - Other

A
Adverse effect of drugs —*see* Table of Drugs and Chemicals
Air pressure
change, rapid
due to residence or long visit at high altitude W94.11-
During
ascent (moving upward) (in, from) W94.29-
aircraft W94.23-
underground W94.22-
water W94.21-
descent (moving downward) (in, from) W94.39-
aircraft W94.31-
other descent W94.39-
water W94.32-
high, prolonged W94.0-
low, prolonged W94.12-
Alpine sickness W94.11-
Altitude sickness W94.11-
Anaphylactic shock, anaphylaxis – see Table of Drugs and Chemicals
Arachnidism, arachnoidism X58-
Asphyxia, asphyxiation (by) (from) (due to)
fire —*see* Exposure, fire
food (bone) (seed) - *see* categories T17 and T18
gas —*see* Table of Drugs and Chemicals
vomitus T17.81-
Aspiration
food (any type) (into respiratory tract) (with asphyxia, obstruction respiratory tract, suffocation) – *see* categories T17 and T18
foreign body - *see* Foreign body
vomitus (with aspiration, obstruction respiratory tract, suffocation) T17.81-
Avalanche – see Forces of Nature

B
Bean in nose - *see* categories T17 and T18
Bed set on fire NEC —*see* Exposure, fire, uncontrolled, building, bed
Bends - s*ee* Air, pressure, change
Bite, bitten by
animal - *see* Contact with, animal
human being W50.3-
during/caused by a crowd or human stampede (with fall) W52-
Blizzard X37.2-
Breakage (part of)
ladder (causing fall) W11-
scaffolding (causing fall) W12-
Broken
glass, contact with —*see* Contact, with, glass
power line (causing electric shock) W85-
Bumping against, into – *see* Fall or Striking against

List intent/cause codes before other External Cause codes. Use more than one code if needed to completely explain the circumstances. **Use these codes throughout treatment with applicable 7th character.**

ACCIDENTS - Other

B (continued)
Burn, burned, burning – (due to contact with hot object) *see also* Contact, with, or Exposure, Fire
acid NEC —*see* Table of Drugs and Chemicals
air X14.1-
inhalation of hot air X14.0-
bed, due to cigarette X08.01
bed linen —*see* Exposure, fire, uncontrolled, in building, Bed
blowtorch X08.8 (with ignition) (sets on fire) – if ignition of clothes, *see* Burn, clothing
candle X08.8- - if ignition of clothes, *see* Burn, clothing
caustic liquid, substance (external) (internal) NEC – *see* Table of Drugs and Chemicals
chemical (external) (internal) —*see* War operations or Table of Drugs and Chemicals
cigar (s) or cigarette(s) X08.8 – (causing fire in/on)
bed X08.01-
clothes – see Burn, clothes
furniture X08.21
sofa X08.11
clothes, clothing NEC (from controlled fire) X06.2-
with conflagration —*see* Exposure, fire, uncontrolled, building
ignition (set on fire) clothing NEC X06.2-
nightwear X05-
cooker (hot) X15.8-
drink X10.0-
electric blanket X16-
engine (hot) X17-
fat and cooking oil X10.2-
fire, flames —*see* Exposure, fire
flare, Very pistol —*see* Discharge, firearm NEC
fluid NEC X12-
food X10.1-
furniture X08.2-
due to cigarette X08.21
gases X14.1-
inhalation of hot gases X14.0-
heating appliance X16-
hotplate X15.2-
household appliance NEC X15.8-

B (continued)
Burn, burned, burning - *see also* Exposure, fire (continued)
iron X15.8-
kettle X15.8-
lamp X08.8-
light bulb X15.8-
lighter (cigar) (cigarette) X08.8-
lightning – *see* category T75.0-
liquid NEC (boiling) X12-
machinery X17-
matches X08.8-
metal (molten) (liquid) NEC X18-
object (not producing fire or flames) X19-
oil (cooking) X10.2-
pipe(s) X16-
radiator X16-
saucepan (glass) (metal) X15.3-
skillet X15.3-
sofa, due to cigarette X08.11
steam X13.1-
stove (kitchen) X15.0-
substance NEC X19-
caustic or corrosive NEC – *see* Table of Drugs and Chemicals
toaster X15.1-
tool X17-
vapor X13.1-
vehicle – *see* Accident, transport, nontraffic or traffic by type of vehicle
water (boiling) – X12
watercraft (onboard) – see Accident, transport, Watercraft
Butted by animal – *see* Contact, with, animal, specific animal, struck by

These codes are for <u>accidental</u> injuries. Do not use if injury due to military or war operations, legal intervention, complication or misadventure.

Accidents, Other – Car sickness-Contact with

ACCIDENTS - Other

C
Car sickness T75.3-
Cat – *see* Contact, with, animal, cat
Cataclysm, cataclysmic (any injury) NEC – see Forces of Nature
Catching fire —*see* Exposure, fire
Caught
Between
objects W23-
folding W23.0-
moving W23.0-
stationary W23.1-
sliding door and door frame W23.0-
by, in
machinery (moving parts of) — *see* Contact, with, by type of machine
washing-machine wringer W23.0-
on fire – *see* Exposure, fire or Burn
under packing crate (due to losing grip) W23.1-
Cave-in caused by cataclysmic earth surface movement or eruption —*see* Landslide
Choked, choking (on) (any object except food or vomitus) *see* categories T17 and T18
food (bone) (seed) - *see* categories T17 and T18
vomitus T17.81-
Cloudburst (any injury) X37.8-
Cold, exposure to (excessive) (extreme) (natural) (place) NEC *see* Exposure, cold
Collapse
building (structure) W20.1-
burning X00.2- or X02.2-
dam or man-made structure (causing earth movement) X36.0-
machinery —*see* Contact, with, by type of machinery *see* Contact, with, by type of machine
Combustion, spontaneous —*see* Ignition

C (continued)
Compression
food (lodged in esophagus) - *see* categories T17 and T18
vomitus (logged in esophagus) T17.81-
Constriction (external) (narrowed) (squeezed)
hair W49.01-
jewelry W49.04-
ring W49.04-
rubber band W49.03-
specified item NEC W49.09-
string W49.02-
thread W49.02-
Contact (with) - *see also* Burn, hot or Exposure to
agricultural machine, including animal-powered W30.1-
combine (harvester) W30.0-
dairy equipment W31.82-
derrick W30.89-
hay W30.2-
grain storage elevator W30.3-
other specified NEC W30.89-
power take-off device W30.1-
reaper W30.0-
thresher W30.0-
transport vehicle
moving – *see* Accident, transport
stationary (not moving) W30.81-

List intent/cause codes before other External Cause codes. Use more than one code if needed to completely explain the circumstances. **Use these codes throughout treatment with applicable 7th character.**

Accidents, Other – Contact with animal

ACCIDENTS - Other

C (continued)

Contact (with) {continued}

- animal **(nonvenomous)** (not poisonous) – *see also* Contact with, animal, venomous (poisonous)
  - alligator W58.09-
    - patient bitten by W58.01-
    - patient crushed by W58.03-
    - patient struck by (hit, knocked down) W58.02-
  - amphibians W62.9- *see also* Contact, with (non-venomous), frogs, toads
  - bee (s) X58-
  - bird NOS W61.99- - *see also* specific bird (macaw, duck, etc.)
    - patient bitten by W61.91-
    - patient struck by (hit, knocked down) W61.92-
  - budgie W61.29
    - patient bitten by W61.21
    - patient struck by (hit, knocked down) W61.22
  - buffalo —*see* Contact, with, animal (non-venomous) hoof stock NEC
  - bull – see Cow
  - camel —*see* Contact, with, animal (non-venomous) hoof stock NEC
  - cat W55.09-
    - patient bitten by W55.01-
    - patient scratched by W55.03-
  - chicken W61.39-
    - patient pecked by W61.33-
    - patient struck by (hit, knocked down) W61.32-
  - cockatiel W61.29
    - patient bitten by W61.21
    - patient struck by (hit, knocked down) W61.22
  - cow W55.29-
    - patient bitten by W55.21-
    - patient struck by (hit, knocked down) W55.22-
  - crocodile W58.19-
    - patient bitten by W58.11-
    - patient crushed by W58.13-
    - patient struck by (hit, knocked down) W58.12-
  - deer —*see* Contact, with, animal (nonvenomous) hoof stock NEC

C (continued)

Contact (with) - *see also* Burn, hot or Exposure to

- animal **(nonvenomous)** (not poisonous) - *see also* Contact, animal, venomous (poisonous) (continued)
  - dog W54.8-
    - patient bitten by W54.0-
    - patient struck by (hit, knocked down) W54.1
  - dolphin W56.09-
    - patient bitten by W56.01-
    - patient struck by (hit, knocked down) W56.02-
  - donkey—*see* Contact, with, animal (non-venomous) hoof stock NEC
  - duck W61.69-
    - patient bitten by W61.61-
    - patient struck by (hit, knocked down) W61.62-
  - feces —*see* Contact, with, animal (nonvenomous) specific animal
  - fish W56.59-
    - patient bitten by W56.51-
    - patient struck by (hit) W56.52-
  - frog W62.0- (any contact)
  - giraffe —*see* Contact, with, animal (non-venomous) hoof stock NEC
  - goat – *see* Contact, with, animal (nonvenomous) hoof stock, NEC
  - goose W61.59-
    - patient bitten by W61.51-
    - patient struck by (hit) (knocked down) W61.52-
  - hoof stock NEC (includes buffalo, camel, deer, donkey, giraffe, goat, llama, sheep, zebra) W55.39-
    - patient bitten by W55.31-
    - patient struck by (hit, knocked down) W55.32-

These codes are for <u>accidental</u> injuries. Do not use if injury due to military or war operations, legal intervention, complication or misadventure.

Accidents, Other – Contact with animal (continued)

ACCIDENTS - Other

C (continued)
Contact (with) (continued)
animal **(nonvenomous)** (not poisonous) - *see also* Contact, animal, venomous (poisonous)
horse W55.19 – *see also* Accident, transport, non-traffic or traffic, horse rider or horse-drawn vehicle
patient bitten by W55.11-
patient struck by (hit) (knocked down) W55.12-
insect NEC (any contact) W57-
lizard W59.09-
patient bitten by W59.01-
patient struck by (hit) W59.02-
llama —*see* Contact, with, animal (nonvenomous) hoof stock NEC
macaw W61.19-
patient bitten by W61.11-
patient struck by (hit) W61.12-
mammal (feces) (urine) NOS W55.89 – *see also* Contact, with animal (nonvenomous), specific animal
patient bitten by W55.81-
patient struck by (hit, knocked down) W55.82-
marine animal NEC W56.89 – *see also* Contact, with animal (nonvenomous) specific animal
patient bitten by W56.81-
patient struck by (hit, knocked down) W56.82-
mouse W53.09-
patient bitten by W53.01-
orca (killer whale) W56.29-
patient bitten by W56.21-
patient struck by (hit, knocked down) W56.22-
parrot W61.09-
patient bitten by W61.01-
patient struck by (hit) W61.02-
pig W55.49-
patient bitten by W55.41-
patient struck by (hit, knocked down) W55.42-
psittacine (bird) W61.29
patient bitten by W61.21
patient struck by W61.22
raccoon W55.59-
patient bitten by W55.51-
patient struck by (hit, knocked down) W55.52-
rat W53.19-
patient bitten by W53.11-

C (continued)
Contact (with) (continued)
animal **(nonvenomous)** (not poisonous) - *see also* Contact, animal, venomous (poisonous)
reptile W59.89 - *see also* Contact, with, animal, (nonvenomous) specific animal
patient bitten by W59.81-
patient crushed by W59.83-
patient struck by (hit) W59.82-
rodent NEC (feces) (urine) W53.89- *see also* Contact, with, animal (nonvenomous) mouse, rat or squirrel
patient bitten by W53.81-
sea lion W56.19-
patient bitten by W56.11-
patient struck by (hit) W56.12-
shark W56.49-
patient bitten by W56.41-
patient struck by (hit) W56.42-
sheep – see Contact, with, animal (nonvenomous), hoof stock
snake W59.19–
patient bitten by W59.11-
patient crushed by W59.13-
patient struck by W59.12-
squirrel W53.29-
patient bitten by W53.21-
toad (any contact) W62.1-
tortoise W59.89- *see* Contact, with, turtle
turkey W61.49-
patient pecked by W61.43-
patient struck by (hit, knocked down) W61.42-
turtle W59.29-
sea turtle W59.29-
patient bitten by W59.21-
patient struck by (hit) W59.22-
terrestrial (land) turtle W59.89-
patient bitten by W59.81-
patient crushed by W59.83-
patient struck by (hit) W59.82-
zebra —*see* Contact, with, animal, hoof stock NEC
animal **(venomous)** (poisonous) (any animal) (includes hornet, rattlesnake, cobra, scorpion, etc.) X58-

List intent/cause codes before other External Cause codes. Use more than one code if needed to completely explain the circumstances. **Use these codes throughout treatment with Applicable 7th character.**

ACCIDENTS - Other

C (continued)	C (continued)
Contact (with) see also Burn, hot or Exposure to (continued)	**Contact (with)** - see also Burn, hot or Exposure to (continued)
arrow W21.89-	drill (powered) W29.8-
not thrown, projected or falling W45.8-	earth (land) (seabed) W31.0-
auger W27.0-	metal drill W31.1-
axe W27.0-	nonpowered W27.8-
band-saw (industrial) (used in business) W31.2-	drive belt (nonagricultural) W24.0-
bayonet —see Bayonet wound	dry ice —see Exposure, cold, man-made
bench-saw (industrial) (used in business) W31.2-	dryer (clothes) (powered) (spin) (used in home) W29.2-
blender (used in home) W29.0-	commercial (used in business) W31.82-
commercial (used in business) W31.82-	earth (-)
boiling water X12-	drilling machine (industrial) W31.0-
bumper cars W31.81-	scraping machine in stationary use W31.83-
can	electric - see also Contact, with, specific electrical device
lid W26.8-	blanket X16-
opener W27.4-	elevator (in building) (nonagricultural) W24.0-
powered (electric) W29.0-	grain W30.3-
chain	engine (s), hot NEC X17 – see also internal combustion engine
hoist W24.0-	excavating machine W31.0-
saw W29.3-	farm machine – see Contact, with agricultural machine
chisel W27.0-	fan (electric) (commercial) (used in home) W29.2-
circular saw W31.2-	commercial (used in business) W31.82-
clothes dryer – see Dryer	food processor (used in home) W29.0-
conveyer belt W24.1-	commercial (used in business) W31.82-
coral X58-	forging (metalworking) machine W31.1-
cotton gin W31.82-	fork W27.4-
crane (nonagricultural) W24.0-	forklift (truck) (nonagricultural) W24.0-
agricultural W30.89-	garbage disposal (used in home) W29.0-
cultivator W29.3-	commercial (used in business) W31.82-
riding (agricultural) W30.89-	garden (tool) – see also Contact, with, rake, hoe, hedge-trimmer, lawnmower, etc. W29.3-
dagger W26.1-	cultivator (powered) W29.3-
dairy equipment W31.82-	riding (agricultural) W30.89-
dart W21.89-	
not thrown, projected or falling W45.8-	
derrick (nonagricultural) W24.0-	
agricultural W30.89-	
hay W30.2-	
dishwasher (used in home) W29.2-	
commercial (used in business) W31.82-	

Note: These codes are for <u>accidental</u> injuries. Do not use if injury due to military or war operations, legal intervention, complication or misadventure.

Accidents, Other – Contact with, gas turbine to rope

ACCIDENTS - Other

C (continued)
Contact (with) (continued)
- gas turbine W31.3-
- glass (sharp) (broken) W25-
  - with subsequent fall W18.02-
  - due to fall —see Fall, by type
  - fall, with subsequent fall against glass W01.110
- Hand
  - saw W27.0-
  - tool (not powered) NEC W27.8-
- hedge-trimmer (powered) W29.3-
- hoe W27.1-
- hoist (chain) (shaft) NEC (nonagricultural) W24.0-
- hot water (tap) X11.8-
  - boiling X12-
  - heated on stove X12-
  - in bathtub X11.0-
  - running X11.1-
- household appliance, implement, or machine W29.8
- ice maker (domestic) (used in home) W29.0-
  - commercial (used in business) W31.82-
- icepick W27.4-
- internal combustion engine W31.3-
- kitchen appliance W29.0- (used in home) - see also specific appliance – food processor, knife, mixer
  - commercial (used in business) W31.82-
- knife W26.0-
  - electric W29.1-
- lathe (metalworking) W31.1-
  - woodworking W31.2-
- lawnmower (powered) (ridden) W28-
  - causing electrocution W86.8-
  - unpowered (push mower) W27.1-
- lift, lifting (devices) (nonagricultural) W24.0-
- machine, machinery NOS W31.9- see also Contact, specific type of machine
  - specified NEC W31.89-
- meat grinder (domestic) (slicer) (used in home) W29.0-
  - industrial (commercial) (used in business) W31.82-
  - nonpowered W27.4-

C (continued)
Contact (with) (continued)
- merry go round W31.81-
- metalworking (industrial) machine W31.1-
- milling, metal machine W31.1-
- mining machine W31.0-
- mixer (domestic) (used in home) W29.0-
  - commercial (used in business) W31.82-
- molding machine W31.2-
- motor – see internal combustion engine
- nail (entering through skin) W45.0-
  - gun W29.4-
- needle (sewing) W27.3- see also Contact with, sewing machine
  - hypodermic W46.0-
    - contaminated W46.1-
- object (blunt) NEC
  - hot NEC X19-
  - sharp NEC W45.8-
- paper (as sharp object) (paper cut) W26.2-
- paper-cutter W27.5-
- pipe, hot X16-
- pitchfork W27.1-
- plane (metal) (wood) W27.0-
  - overhead W31.2-
- plant thorns, spines, sharp leaves (nonvenomous) W60-
  - venomous T63.7-
- power press, metal W31.1-
- prime mover W31.3-
- printer machine W31.89-
- pulley (block) (transmission) W24.0-
  - agricultural W30.89-
- rake W27.1-
- rivet gun (powered) W29.4-
- roller coaster W31.81-
- rope NEC W24.0-
  - agricultural W30.89-

Note: List intent/cause codes before other External Cause codes. Use more than one code if needed to completely explain the circumstances. **Use these codes throughout treatment with applicable 7th character.**

Accidents, Other – Contact with, saliva to Cyclone

ACCIDENTS - Other

C (continued)
Contact (with) - *see also* Burn or Exposure to (cont.)
saliva —*see* Contact, with, by type of animal
sander (used at home) W29.8-
commercial (used in business) W31.82-
saucepan (hot) (glass) (metal) X15.3-
saw W27.0-
band (industrial) W31.2-
bench (industrial) W31.2-
chain (used at home) W29.3-
hand (nonpowered) W27.0-
scissors W27.2-
screwdriver W27.0-
powered W29.8-
sewing-machine (electric) (powered) (used in home) W29.2-
commercial (used in business) W31.82-
not powered W27.8-
shaft (hoist) (lift) (transmission) NEC W24.0-
agricultural W30.89-
shears (hand) W27.2-
domestic (used at home) W29.2-
powered (used in business) W31.1-
shovel (nonpowered) W27.8-
skillet (hot) X15.3-
spade W27.1-
spinning machine W31.89-
splinter W45.8-
sports equipment NOS W21.9- *see also* specific sports equipment
staple gun (powered) W29.8-
steam X13.1-
engine W31.3-
inhalation X13.0-
pipe X16-
shovel W31.89-
stove (hot) (kitchen) X15.0-
substance, hot NEC X19-
molten (melted) (metal) X18-
sword W26.1-
toaster (hot) X15.1-
tool W27.8- *see also* specific tool (axe, chisel, saw)
hand (not powered) W27.8 - *see also* specific tool (garden, kitchen, workbench)
auger W27.0-
specified NEC W27.8-
hot X17-
powered W29.8-

C (continued)
Contact (with) - *see also* Burn or Exposure to (continued)
transmission device (belt, cable, chain, gear, pinion, shaft) W24.1-
turbine (gas) (water-driven) W31.3-
under-cutter W31.0-
urine —*see* Contact, with, by type of animal
vehicle - *see* Accident, transport
washing machine (used at home) W29.2-
commercial (used in business) W31.82-
weaving-machine W31.89-
winch W24.0-
agricultural W30.89-
wood slivers W45.8-
workbench W27.0-
Corrosive liquid, substance —*see* Table of Drugs and Chemicals
Crash – transport vehicle NEC – *see* Accident, transport
Crushed X58-
between objects (moving) W23.0-
stationary W23.1-
by
animal – *see* Contact, with, animal, venomous or non-venomous, specific animal
avalanche NEC —*see* Landslide
cave-in W20.0-
caused by cataclysmic earth surface movement- *see* Landslide
crowd or human stampede W52-
falling (falling object hit patient) (falling from)
aircraft (patient on ground) V97.39-
earth, material W20.0-
caused by cataclysmic earth surface movement – *see* Landslide
object NEC W20.8-
landslide NEC —*see* Landslide
machinery —*see* Contact, with, by type of machine
Cut, cutting (any part of body) – *see* Contact, with, by object or machine
Cyclone (any injury) X37.1-

Note: These codes are for accidental injuries. Do not use if injury due to military or war operations, legal intervention, complication or misadventure.

Accidents, Other – Decapitation to Drowning/submersion

ACCIDENTS - Other

D	D (continued)
Decapitation (accidental) NEC X58-	**Drowning and submersion** W74- (in) (continued)
Dehydration from lack of water X58-	bucket (fall into) W16.221-
Deprivation X58-	due to
Desertion X58-	cloudburst X37.8-
Destitution X58-	cyclone X37.1-
Derailment - *see* Accident, transport, nontraffic or traffic, by type of vehicle	fall overboard (from) -- *see* Accident, transport, watercraft
Discharge	jumping into water from watercraft (involved in accident) - *see* Accident, transport, watercraft V90.89-
firearm W34.00–*see also* Malfunction, firearm	tidal wave NEC —*see* Forces of nature, tidal wave
air gun W34.010-	torrential rain X37.8-
BB gun W34.010-	fountain —*see* Drowning or submersion, following, fall, into, water, specified NEC
flare gun W34.09-	natural water (lake) (open sea) (river) (stream) (pond) W69-
gas-operated gun NEC W34.018-	without fall W69-
handgun (pistol) (revolver) W32.0-	dive or jump W16.611-
hunting rifle W33.02-	striking bottom W16.621-
machine gun W33.03-	fall (into water) W16.111-
paintball gun W34.011-	striking bottom W16.121-
pellet gun W34.010-	striking side W16.131-
shotgun W33.01-	quarry —*see* Drowning or submersion, following, fall, into,
specified NEC W34.09-	reservoir —*see* Drowning or submersion, following, fall, into, water, specified NEC
spring-operated gun NEC W34.018-	river —*see* Drowning or Submersion, in, natural water
Very pistol (flare gun) W34.09-	sea —*see* Drowning or Submersion, in, natural water
firework(s) W39-	specified place NEC W73 (following)
Diving —*see* Jumped, Fall, into, water	dive or jump W16.811-
with drowning or submersion– see Drowning and submersion	striking bottom W16.821-
Dragged by transport vehicle NEC (pedestrian on foot or using conveyance) *see also* Accident, transport V09.9-	striking wall W16.831-
	fall (into water NEC) W16.311-
Drinking poison (accidental) – *see* Table of Drugs and Chemicals	striking bottom W16.821-
	striking wall W16.831-
Dropped while being carried or supported by other person W04-	swimming pool W16.011-
	dive or jump W16.511-
Drowning or submersion (in) W74- (in) *see also* Fall, water	striking bottom W16.521-
	striking wall W16.531-
bathtub	fall (into pool) W16.011-
fall in bathtub W65-	striking bottom W16.021-
fall into bathtub W16.211-	striking wall W16.031-
boat (jump or dive from) W16.711-	water NOS (fall into) W16.41-
striking bottom W16.721-	

Note: List intent/cause codes before other External Cause codes. Use more than one code if needed to completely explain the circumstances. **Use these codes throughout treatment with applicable 7th character.**

ACCIDENTS - Other

E	E (continued)
Earth falling (on) W20.0-	**Explosion (of)** (with secondary fire) W40.9 (continued)
caused by cataclysmic earth surface movement or eruption - *see* Landslide	gas (coal) (explosive) W40.1-
Earthquake (any injury) X34-	aerosol can W36.1-
Effect(s) (adverse) of	air tank W36.2-
air pressure (any) —*see* Air, pressure	cylinder W36.9-
cold, excessive (exposure to) —*see* Exposure, cold	fumes W40.1-
heat (excessive) —*see* Heat	pressurized gas tank W36.3-
hot place (weather) —*see* Heat	specified NEC W36.8-
late —*see* Sequelae	gasoline (fumes) (tank) not in moving motor vehicle W40.1-
radiation —*see* Radiation	bomb W40.8-
Electric	in motor vehicle —*see* Accident, transport
current —*see* Exposure, electric current	grenade W40.8-
motor - *see also* Contact, with, by type of machine W31-	hose, pressurized W37.8-
	hot water heater, tank (in machinery) W35-
Electrocution (accidental) —*see* Exposure, electric	on watercraft —*see* Explosion, in, watercraft
Entanglement (in)	in
bed linen, causing suffocation —*see* category T71-	dump W40.8-
wheel of pedal cycle V19.88-	factory W40.8-
Environmental factor NEC X58-	grain store W40.8-
Environmental pollution related condition Z57-	mine W40.1-
Exhaustion – *see also* Overexertion	munitions (dump) (factory) W40.8-
cold —*see* Exposure, cold	letter bomb W40.8-
due to excessive exertion —*see* category X50-	machinery —*see also* Contact, with, by type of machine
heat —*see* Heat	on board watercraft V93.59- *see also* Accident, watercraft
Explosion (of) (with secondary fire) W40.9-	pressure vessel —*see* Explosion, by type of vessel
acetylene W40.1-	methane W40.1-
aerosol can W36.1-	missile NEC W40.8-
air tank (compressed) (in machinery) W.36.2-	mortar bomb W40.8-
aircraft (in transit) (powered) – see Accident, transport, aircraft	munitions (dump) (factory) W40.8-
	pipe, pressurized W37.8-
anesthetic gas in operating room W40.1-	bomb W40.8-
bicycle tire W37.0-	pressure, pressurized
blasting (cap) (materials) W40.0-	cooker W38-
boiler (machinery), not on transport vehicle W35-	gas tank (in machinery) W36.3-
on watercraft —*see* Accident, transport, watercraft	hose W37.8-
butane W40.1-	specified device NEC W38-
coal gas W40.1-	vessel (in machinery) W38-
detonator W40.0-	propane W40.1-
dynamite W40.0-	shell (artillery) NEC W40.8-
explosive (material) W40.9-	spacecraft V95.45-
gas (fumes) W40.1-	steam or water lines (in machinery) W37.8-
in blasting operation W40.0-	tire, pressurized (vehicle) W37.8-
specified NEC W40.8-	bicycle W37.0-
fertilizer bomb W40.8-	watercraft (powered) V93.59- *see also* Accident, transport, watercraft
firearm (parts) NEC W34.19- *see also* Discharge, firearm or Malfunction, firearm	
fireworks W39-	

These codes are used for <u>accidental</u> injuries. Do not use if injury due to military or war operations, legal intervention, or medical treatment/complication.

Accidents, Other – Exposure to, cold to electrical current

ACCIDENTS - Other

E (continued)
Exposure (to) - *see also* Contact with
cold (excessive) (extreme) (natural) (due to) X31-
man-made conditions W93.8-
dry ice (contact with) W93.01-
inhalation W93.02-
liquid air (contact) (hydrogen) (nitrogen) W93.11-
inhalation W93.12-
refrigeration unit (deep freeze) W93.2-
weather (conditions) X31-
electric current W86.8-
appliance (faulty) W86.8-
domestic (used in home) W86.0-
conductor (faulty) W86.1-
control apparatus (faulty) W86.1-
electric power generating plant, distribution station W86.1-
high-voltage cable (broken) W85-

E (continued)
Exposure (to) - *see also* Contact with (continued)
electric current W86.8- (continued)
in
home (wiring) (appliances) W86.0-
public building (wiring) (appliances) W86.8-
residential institution (wiring) (appliances) W86.8-
schools (wiring) (appliances) W86.8-
lightning —*see* subcategory T75.0-
live rail W86.8-
motor (electric) (faulty) W86.8-
domestic (used in home) W86.0-
on farm (not including farmhouse) W86.8-
outdoors (wiring) (appliances) W86.8-
specified NEC W86.8-
domestic (used in home) W86.0-
taser (stun gun) W86.8-
third rail W86.8-
taser (stun gun) W86.8-
transformer (faulty) W86.1-
transmission lines (broken) W85-
environmental tobacco smoke X58-

List intent/cause codes before other External Cause codes. Use more than one code if needed To completely explain the circumstances.
Use these codes throughout treatment with applicable 7th character.

These codes are used for <u>accidental</u> injuries. Do not use if injury is due to military or war operations, legal intervention or medical treatment/complication.

ACCIDENTS, Other

E (continued)
Exposure (to) - *see also* Contact with
fire, flames X08.8 – *see also* Burn
controlled fire – *see also* Unspecified fires, Uncontrolled fire
in building or structure (with) (resulting in) X02.0-
fall from building X02.3-
hit by object from building X02.4-
injury due to building collapse X02.2-
jump from building X02.5-
other specified injury X02.8-
not in building or structure (with) X03.0-
fall X03.3-
hit by object X03.4-
smoke inhalation X03.1-
other specified injury NEC X03.8-
other specified injury X02.8-
uncontrolled fire – *see also* Controlled fire, Unspecified fire
in building or structure (with) (resulting in) X00.3-
hit by object from building X00.4-
injury due to building collapse X00.2-
jump from building X00.5-
other specified injury X00.8-
not in building or structure (with) X01.0-
fall X01.3-
hit by object X01.4-
smoke inhalation X01.1-
other specified injury NEC X01.8-

E (continued)
Exposure (to) - *see also* Contact with
fire, flames X08.8 – *see also* Burn
unspecified (other) fire – *see also* Controlled and Uncontrolled fire (in) (on) (started in)
bed (mattress) (due to) X08.00-
cigarette X08.01-
specified material NEC X08.09-
clothing and apparel X06.2-
nightwear X05-
furniture NEC (due to) X08.20-
cigarette X08.21-
other specific material NEC X08.29-
sofa (due to) X08.10-
highly flammable materials X04-
gasoline X04-
kerosene X04-
machinery – *see* Contact, with, by type of machine
melting (due to fire)
clothing and apparel X06.3-
nightwear X05-
plastic jewelry X06.1-
plastic jewelry X06.0-
melted (melting) X06.1-
resulting from
explosion —*see* Explosion
lightning X08.8-
sofa (due to) X08.10-
transport vehicle – *see* Accident, nontraffic or Traffic

Controlled fire – Fire or flame deliberately started for benign purpose (such as for cooking or providing heat). Examples are: campfire, bonfire, trash fire, in fireplace or stove. See X02-X03.

Uncontrolled fire – Fire or flame accidentally started (such as fire in building or forest, caught on fire by cigarette). See X00-X01

Unspecified (other) fire – Fire not documented as controlled or uncontrolled. Includes other fires, such as clothing or furniture fires. See X04-X08

Accidents, Other – Exposure to, forces of nature to wind

ACCIDENTS - Other

E (continued)	E (continued)
Exposure (to) - *see also* Contact with (continued)	**Exposure (to)** - *see also* Contact with (continued)
forces of nature NEC —*see* Forces of nature	radiation —*see* Radiation
heat (natural) NEC —*see* Heat	smoke —*see also* Exposure, fire
lightning —*see* subcategory T75.0-	tobacco, second hand Z77.22
causing fire —*see* Exposure, fire, not in building or structure	specified factors NEC X58-
mechanical forces	sunlight X32-
animate (living, human or animal) NEC W64-	man-made (sun lamp) W89.8-
inanimate NEC (nonliving object or machine) W49.9-	supersonic waves W42.0
	tanning bed W89.1
noise W42.9-	tobacco (smoke) (environmental) X58-
supersonic W42.0-	transmission line(s), electric W85-
	vibration W49.9-
	weather NEC —*see* Forces of nature
	wind NEC – *see* Forces of nature

List intent/cause codes before other External Cause codes. Use more than one code if needed to completely explain The circumstances. **Use these codes throughout treatment with applicable 7th character.**

These codes are used for accidental injuries. Do not use if Injury is due to military or war operations, legal intervention Or medical treatment/complication.

ACCIDENTS - Other

F

Fall, falling W19- Includes falling down, from, in, into, out, over, through. *See also* Accident, transport, Exposure to fire, Jumped, Pushed, Slipped, Stumbled, or Drowning and submersion

- aircraft – *see* Accident, transport, aircraft
- animal (fell over) W01.0-
- balcony W13.0-
- bed W06-
- bridge W13.1-
- bucket (utility) W16.222-
    - causing drowning or submersion W16.221-
- building W13.9-
    - burning building X00.3- or X02.3-
    - collapsed building W20-
- bumping against (collision with) (followed by fall) – *see also* Striking against
    - object W18.01-
    - person W03-
        - due to ice or snow W00.0-
        - involving pedestrian conveyance – see Accident, transport, traffic or nontraffic
- chair W07-
- cherry picker W17.89-
- cliff W15-
- dock W17.4-
- dropped while being carried or supported by another person W04-
- earth – *see* Earth, falling
- elevated work platform (MEWP) W17.89-
- embankment W17.81-
- escalator W10.0-
- flagpole W13.8-
- floor (fall through) W13.3-
- furniture NEC W08-
- grocery cart (tipping over) W17.82-
- haystack W17.89-
- high place NEC W17.89-
- hill (fall down) W17.81-
- hole W17.2-
- ice or snow W00.9-
    - from one level to another W00.2-
        - on stairs or steps W00.1-
- incline W10.2-
- ladder W11-
- lifting device W17.89-
- machine, machinery – *see also* Contact, with, type of machine
    - not in use W17.89-
- manhole W17.1-
- object, edged, pointed or sharp (with cut)
    - small object (fall over) W01.0-
- on same level W18.3-
    - with subsequent striking against glass W01.110

F (continued)

Fall, falling W19 (due to) (from) (continued)

- one level to another NEC W17.8-
- pit W17.2
- playground equipment W09.8-
    - jungle gym W09.2-
    - slide W09.0-
    - swing W09.1-
- quarry W17.89-
- railing W13.0-
- ramp W10.2-
- rock (fell over) W20.8-
    - thrown W21-
- roof W13.2-
- scaffolding W12-
- shaft W17.89-
- shower W18.2-
    - causing drowning or submersion W16.21-
- sidewalk curb W10.1-
- sky lift W17.89-
- stairs, staircase, steps W10.9-
    - curb W10.1-
    - due to ice or snow W00.1-
    - escalator W10.0-
    - specified NEC W10.8-
- standing (on)
    - electric scooter V00.841
    - micro-mobility pedestrian conveyance V00.848
- stepladder W11-
- stone (fall over) W20.8-
- storm drain W17.1-
- streetcar – *see* Accident, transport, traffic or nontraffic
- structure NEC W13.8-
    - burning (uncontrolled fire) X00.3-
- table W08-
- tank W17.89-
- toilet W18.11- (fall not followed by striking object)
    - followed by striking against object W18.12-
- train - *see also* Accident, transport, traffic or nontraffic
- tree W14-
    - hit by falling tree struck by lightning W20.8-
- vehicle (in motion) – *see also* Accident, transport, traffic or nontraffic
    - while stationary W17.89-
- viaduct W13.8-
- wall W13.8-
- watercraft – *see* Accident, transport, watercraft
- well W17.0-
- wheelchair – *see* Accident, transport, traffic or nontraffic
- window W13.4-
- work platform (elevated) W17.89-

Accidents, Other – Fire to Lost at sea

ACCIDENTS - Other

F (continued)	
Fire —*see* Exposure, fire or Burn	
Firearm discharge —*see* Discharge, firearm	
Fireworks (explosion) W39-	
Flash burns from explosion —*see* Explosion	
Flood (any injury) (caused by) X38-	
	tidal wave —*see* Forces of nature, tidal wave
Food (any type) in	
	air passages (with asphyxia, obstruction, or suffocation) *See* categories T17 and T18
	alimentary (digestive) tract causing asphyxia - *see* categories T17 and T18
Forces of nature X39.8-	
	avalanche X36.1-
		causing transport accident – see Accident, transport, nontraffic or traffic
	blizzard X37.2-
	cataclysmic storm X37.9-
		with flood X38-
	cloudburst X37.8-
	cyclone X37.1-
	dust storm 37.3-
	heat (natural) (causing sunstroke) X30-
	flood (caused by) X38-
		dam collapse X36.0-
		tidal wave —*see* Forces of nature, tidal wave
	hurricane X37.0-
	landslide X36.1-
	lightning —*see* subcategory T75.0-
		causing fire —*see* Exposure, fire
	mudslide X36.1-
	radiation (natural) X39.08-
	radon X39.01-
	snow and ice X37.2-
	specified force NEC X39.8-
	specified storm NEC X37.8-
	storm surge X37.0-
	structure collapse causing earth movement X36.0-
	sunlight X32-
	tidal wave (due to) X37.4-
		earthquake X37.41-
		landslide X37.43-
		storm X37.42-
		volcanic eruption X37.41-
	tornado X37.1-
	tsunami X37.41-
	twister X37.1-
	typhoon X37.0-
	volcanic eruption X35-

K	
Kicked by (animal or person kicked patient) *see also* – Struck by	
	animal – see Contact, with, animal, specific animal, struck by
	person (s) W50.1-
Kicking against (patient kicked object or person) *see also* - Striking against	
	object W22.8-
	sports equipment W21.9-
		specified W21.89-
	stationary object W22.09-
	person —*see* Striking against, person
Killed, killing NOS - *see* Injury X58-	
Knocked down (by) NOS X58-	
	animal (not being ridden) — *see* Contact, with, animal, by type of animal, struck by
	crowd or human stampede W52-
	transport vehicle NEC - *see* Accident, transport, nontraffic or traffic V09.09-

L	
Laceration NEC —*see* Injury	
Lack of	
	care (helpless person) (infant) (newborn) X58-
	food except as result of abandonment or neglect X58-
	water except as result of transport accident X58-
		helpless person, infant, newborn X58-
Landslide (falling on transport vehicle) X36.1-	
Late effect - use code for original injury with 7th character S	
Lifting – *see also* Overexertion	
	heavy objects X50.0-
	weights X50.0-
Lightning (shock) (stroke) (struck by) – see subcategory T75.0-	
	causing fire —*see* Exposure, fire
Loss of control (transport vehicle) – *see* Accident, transport, nontraffic or traffic	
Lost at sea NOS – *see* Drowning or submersion, due to, fall overboard	

These codes are used for <u>accidental</u> injuries. Do not use if injury Is due to military or war operations, legal intervention or medical/complication.

ACCIDENTS - Other

M

Machine, machinery —see Contact, with, by type of machine

Malfunction, gun (mechanism or component) (includes Explosion of) W34.10-
- air gun W34.110-
- BB gun W34.110-
- flare gun W34.19-
- gas gun NEC W34.118-
- handgun W32.1-
- hunting rifle W33.12-
- larger firearm W33.10-
- machine gun W33.13-
- paintball gun W34.111-
- pellet gun W34.110-
- shotgun W33.11-
- specified NEC W34.19-
- spring-operated gun NEC W34.118-
- Very pistol [flare] W34.19-

Mangled NOS X58-

Melting (due to fire) – see Exposure, fire, melting

Motion sickness T75.3-

Mudslide (of cataclysmic nature) – see Landslide

N

Nail, contact with (entering skin) W45.0-
- gun W29.4-

Noise (causing injury) (pollution) W42.9-
- supersonic waves W42.0-

O

Object
- falling – see Fall, falling
- set in motion (started moving due to)
  - explosion or rupture of pressure vessel W38-
  - firearm – see Discharge, firearm, by type
  - machine(ry) – see Contact, with, by type of machine

Overdose (drug) —see also Table of Drugs and Chemicals
- during treatment – see Complications

Overexertion (from) X50.9-
- prolonged static or awkward postures X50.1-
- repetitive movement X50.3-
- specified strenuous movements or postures NEC X50.9-
- strenuous movements or load X50.0-

Overexposure – see Exposure (to)

Overheated —see Heat

Overturning
- machinery —see Contact, with, by type of machine
- transport vehicle NEC - see also Accident, transport, nontraffic or traffic V89.9-
- watercraft (causing drowning or submersion) – see Drowning or submersion, due to, accident, to, watercraft

P

Parachute – see Accident, transport, aircraft, nonpowered

Piercing —see Contact, with, by type of object or machine

Pinched – see Caught or Crushed

Pinned under machine(ry) —see Contact, with, by type of machine

Poisoning (by) —see also Table of Drugs and Chemicals
- carbon monoxide (exhaust fumes) (generated by)
  - fumes or smoke due to
    - explosion (see also Explosion) W40.1-
    - fire – see Exposure, fire
    - motor vehicle —see Accident, transport, nontraffic, or traffic
  - watercraft – see Accident, transport, watercraft
- marine or sea plants (venomous) (poisonous) X58-
- plant, thorns, spines, sharp leaves NEC X58-

Powder burn (by) (from) – see Accident, discharge or Malfunction, firearm

Prolonged (stay in)
- high altitude as cause of anoxia, barodontalgia, barotitis or hypoxia W94.11-
- weightless environment X52-

Pulling, excessive —see category Y93-

Pushed, pushing (injury in) – see Fall

List intent/cause codes before other External Cause codes. Use more Than one code if needed to completely explain the circumstances. **Use these codes throughout treatment with applicable 7th character.**

Accidents, Other – Radiation to Steam

ACCIDENTS - Other

R
Radiation (exposure to)
arc lamps W89.0-
atomic power plant (malfunction) NEC W88.1-
electromagnetic, ionizing W88.0-
gamma rays W88.1-
infrared (heaters and lamps) W90.1-
excessive heat from W92-
man-made visible light W89.9
specified NEC W89.8-
tanning bed W89.1-
ultraviolet (light) W89.8-
welding arc, torch, or light W89.0-
excessive heat from W92-
microwave W90.8-
natural light source NEC X39.08-
sunlight X32-
ultraviolet X32-
radar W90.0-
radiofrequency W90.0-
radioisotopes W88.1-
radium NEC W88.1-
specified NEC W88.8-
x-rays (hard) (soft) W88.0-
Recoil – Firearm – *see* Discharge or Malfunction, firearm
Rock falling on or hitting (person) W20.8-
in cave-in W20.0-
Run over (by)
animal
being ridden – *see* Accident, transport, nontraffic or traffic, animal
not being ridden – *see* Contact with, animal, specific, animal, struck by
transport vehicle NEC - *see* Accident, transport, nontraffic or traffic
Running off, away
Animal
being ridden – *see* Accident, transport, nontraffic or traffic, animal
not being ridden – *see* Contact with, animal, specific animal, struck by
on highway or road – *see* Accident, transport, nontraffic or traffic

S
Scratched by
animal – *see* Contact, with, animal, specific animal
person (s) (accidentally) W50.4-
Scald, scalding – *see* Burn
Seasickness T75.3-
Sequelae – use code for original injury with 7th character S
Shock (electric) – *see* Exposure, electric current
Shooting, shot —*see* Discharge, firearm, by type
Sinking watercraft – *see* Accident, transport, watercraft
Slipping (on same level) (with fall) (includes Tripping) *see also* Accident, transport, Fall, Jumped, or Stumbling
with subsequent striking against glass W01.110
without fall (due to) W18.40-
specified NEC W18.49-
stepping from one level to another W18.43-
stepping into hole or opening W18.42-
stepping on object W18.41-
fall without striking object W01.0-
on
ice W00.0-
on skates – *see* Accident, transport, skates
mud W01.0-
oil W01.0-
snow W00.0-
on skis – *see* Accident, transport, skis
surface (slippery) (wet) NEC W01.0-
over animal W01.0-
Sound waves (causing injury) W42.9-
supersonic waves W42.0-
Splinter, contact with W45.8-
Stab, stabbing —*see* Cut
Starvation X58-
Steam X13.1-
inhalation X13.0-
pipe X16-

These codes are used for <u>accidental</u> injuries. Do not use for Injures due to military or war operations, legal intervention or medical treatment/complications.

ACCIDENTS - Other

S

Stepped on (by) (animal or person stepped on patient) – see also Stepping on, Striking against
- animal (not being ridden) – see Contact, animal, by specific animal
- crowd or human stampede W52-
- person W50.0-

Stepping on (patient stepped on object or person) – see also Stepped on, Striking against
- object W22.8-
  - with fall W18.31-
  - stationary object W22.09-
- person W51-
  - by crowd or human stampede W52-
- sports equipment W21.9-
  - specified NEC W21.89

Strangulation (accidental) —see category T71-

Strenuous movements —see category Y93-

Striking against (patient hit object or person) (includes walking into) – see also Struck by, Kicked against
- after falling into water – see Drowning or submersion
- airbag (automobile) W22.10-
  - driver side W22.11-
  - front passenger side W22.12-
  - specified NEC W22.19-
- furniture W22.03-
- lamppost W22.02-
- object (with) W22.8-
  - caused by crowd or human stampede (with fall) W52-
  - stationary object W22.09-
- person (s) W51-
  - with fall W03-
    - due to ice or snow W00.0-
    - due to crowd or human stampede (with fall) W52-
- sports equipment W21.9-
  - specified NEC W21.89-
- wall W22.01- see also Jumping or Falling, into water

Struck by (object or person hit patient)-see also Striking against
- animal
  - being ridden – see Accident, transport, nontraffic or traffic, animal-rider
  - not being ridden – see Contact, with, animal, struck by or Accident, transport, nontraffic or traffic, animal

List intent/cause codes before other External Cause codes. Use more than one code if needed to completely explain the circumstances. **Use these codes throughout treatment with applicable 7th character.**

S (continued)

Struck by (object or person hit patient) (continued)
- ball (hit by) (thrown) W21.09-
  - baseball W21.03-
  - basketball W21.05-
  - football W21.01-
  - golf ball W21.04-
  - soccer W21.02-
  - softball W21.07-
  - volleyball W21.06-
- bat or racquet (club) W21.19-
  - baseball bat W21.11-
  - golf club W21.13-
  - tennis racquet W21.12-
- bullet —see Discharge, firearm by type
- hailstones X39.8-
- hockey
  - field hockey
    - puck W21.221-
    - stick W21.211-
  - ice hockey
    - puck W21.220-
    - stick W21.210-
- lightning —see subcategory T75.0-
  - causing fire —see Exposure, fire
- machine (in operation) —see Contact, with, by machine
- object (blunt) (on) W22.8
  - falling (object fell from or due to) W20.8-
    - building (object fell from) W20.1-
      - burning X00.4-
      - collapsing building (on fire) X00.2
    - set in motion by explosion – see Explosion W20.8-
- other person (s) (with) W50.0-
- structure (collapsing) W20.1-
  - burning X00.2-
  - due to crowd or human stampede (with fall) W52-
  - blunt object W22.8-
  - fall W03-
    - due to ice or snow W00.0-
- sports equipment W21.9-
  - cleats (shoe) W21.31-
  - football helmet W21.81-
  - skate blades W21.32-
  - specified NEC W21.89-
- thunderbolt —see subcategory T75.0-
  - causing fire —see Exposure, fire
- transport vehicle (in motion) — see Accident, transport, nontraffic or traffic
- watercraft – see Accident, transport, watercraft

Accidents, Other – Stumbling to Work related condition

ACCIDENTS - Other

S (continued)	
Stumbling – *see also* Accident, transport, Fall, Jumped, or Slipping	
	without fall (due to) W18.40-
	specified NEC W18.49-
	stepping from one level to another W18.43-
	stepping on object W18.41-
	Over
	animal NEC W01.0-
	with fall W18.09-
	carpet or rug W22.8-
	with fall W18.09-
	object (small) W22.8-
	with fall W18.09-
	person (without fall) W51-
	with fall W03-
	due to ice and snow W00.0-
Submersion —*see* Drowning or submersion	
Suffocation (by external means) (by pressure) (mechanical) (due to) *see also category T71*)	
	avalanche —*see* Landslide
	burning building X00.8-, X02.8-
	explosion —*see* Explosion
	fire —*see* Exposure, fire
	food, any type (aspiration) (ingestion) (inhalation) – see categories T17 and T18
	landslide —*see* Landslide
	machine (ry) —*see* Contact, with, by type of Machine
	vomitus (aspiration) (inhalation) T17.81-
Sunstroke X32-	
Supersonic waves W42.0-	
Swallowed, swallowing	
	caustic or corrosive substance —*see* Table of Drugs and Chemicals
	foreign body —*see* category T18-
	poison —*see* Table of Drugs and Chemicals

T	
Tackle in sport W03-	
Thirst X58-	
Thrown (from) (off)	
	machinery – *see* Contact, with, by type of machine
	transport vehicle – *see* Accident, transport, nontraffic or traffic
Thunderbolt —*see* subcategory T75.0-	
	causing fire —*see* Exposure, fire
Tidal wave (any injury) NEC —*see* Forces of nature, tidal wave	
Tornado (any injury) X37.1-	
Torrential rain (any injury) X37.8-	
Trampled by animal NEC W55.89- *see also* Contact, with, animal	
	transport vehicle – *see* Accident, transport, nontraffic or traffic
Trapped (accidentally)	
	between objects (moving) (stationary and moving) - *see also* Caught by part (any) of
	motorcycle V29.88-
	pedal cycle V19.88-
	transport vehicle NEC - *see also* Accident, transport V89.9-
Travel (effects) (sickness) T75.3-	
Tree falling on or hitting (person) W20.8-	
Tripping - see Slipping	
Twisted by person (s) W50.2-	
	as, or caused by, a crowd or human stampede (with fall) W52-
V	
Vibration (causing injury) W49.9-	
Volcanic eruption (any injury) X35-	
Vomitus, gastric contents in air passages (with asphyxia, obstruction or suffocation) T17.81-	
W	
Walked into stationary object (any) – *see* Striking Against	
Washed	
	away by flood —*see* Flood
	off road by storm (transport vehicle) —*see* Forces of nature, cataclysmic storm
	overboard – *see* Transport, accident, watercraft
Weather exposure NEC —*see* Forces of nature	
Wound (accidental) NEC - *see also* Injury X58-	
Weightlessness (causing injury) (effects of) (in spacecraft, real or simulated) X52-	
Work related condition Y99.0-	

These codes are used for <u>accidental</u> injuries.

Do not use if injury due to military or war operations, legal intervention or medical treatment/complication.

CATEGORY – INTENT/CAUSE - NONACCIDENTS
Assault

A
Abandonment X58-
Abuse (child) (mental) (physical) (sexual) X58-
Appliance (hot) X98.3-
Arson X97-
Asphyxia, asphyxiation
by
food (bone) (seed) – see categories T17 and T18
gas – see Table of Drugs and Chemicals
legal execution – see Legal, intervention, gas
from
fire- see Exposure, fire or Burn
ignition – see Exposure, fire or Burn
vomitus T17.81-
Assassination (attempt) NOS Y09
B
Bite, bitten by (person) (in fight) Y04.1-
Bayonet wound W26.1-
Battered (baby) (child) (person) (syndrome) X58-
Blowing up —see Explosion
Blunt object Y00-
Bodily force Y04.8-
bite Y04.1-
brawl (unarmed) Y04.0-
bumping into Y04.2-
sexual assault - see subcategories T74.0- or T76.0-
Bomb X96.9 – see also Military operations, Operations of war
antipersonnel X96.0-
fertilizer bomb X96.3-
gasoline bomb X96.1-
incendiary device X97-
letter bomb X96.2-
mortar X96.8-
pipe bomb X96.4-
specified NEC X96.8-
Brawl (hand) (fists) (foot) (unarmed) Y04.0-
Bumped into by other person Y04.2
Burning, burns (by fire) NEC X97-
acid Y08.89-
caustic, corrosive substance Y08.89-
chemical from swallowing caustic, corrosive substance —see Table of Drugs and Chemicals
cigarette (s) X97-
hot object X98.8-
fluid NEC X98.2-
household appliance X98.3-
specified NEC X98.8-
steam X98.0-
tap water X98.1-

C
Caustic, corrosive substance (gas) Y08.89-
Crash – see also Run over (by)
aircraft (in transit) (powered) Y08.81-
motor vehicle Y03.8- – see also Accident, transport
pushed in front of Y02.0-
run over V03.0-
specified NEC Y03.8-
Cutting or piercing instrument X99.9-
dagger X99.2-
glass X99.0-
knife X99.1-
specified NEC X99.8-
sword X99.2-
D
Dagger X99.2-
Decapitation X99.9-
Discharge (firearm) X95.9-
air gun X95.01-
BB gun X95.01-
flare X95.8-
gas-operated gun X95.09-
gun NEC — X95.09-
handgun (pistol) (revolver) X93-
hunting rifle X94.1-
machine gun X94.2-
paintball gun X95.02-
pellet gun X95.01-
pistol X93-
revolver X93-
spring-operated gun NEC X95.09-
shotgun X94.0-
specified NEC X95.8-
spring-operated gun NEC X95.09-
Very pistol (flare) X95.8-
Drowning or submersion (patient in) X92.9-
bathtub X92.0-
natural water X92.3-
specified place NEC X92.8-
swimming pool (fall) X92.1-
pushed (into) X92.2-
watercraft (pushed from or off) X92.3-
Dynamite X96.8-

List intent/cause codes before other External Cause codes. Use more than one code if needed to completely explain the circumstances. **Use these codes throughout treatment with applicable 7th character.**

Nonaccidents, Assault, Explosion to Perpetrator

NONACCIDENTS, Assault

E

Explosion – *see also* Bomb
- dynamite X96.8-
- fertilizer bomb X96.3-
- gasoline (fumes) (tank) (not in moving motor vehicle) X96.1-
- grenade X96.8-

Exposure (to) X58-
- cold X58-
- due to abandonment or neglect X58-
- electric current Y08.89-
- fire, flames X97-
- taser Y08.89-

F

Fight (hand) (fists) (foot) (unarmed) Y04.0-
- with weapon —*see* Assault, by type of weapon

Fire X97-

Firearm – *see* Discharge, firearm

Fluids (hot) X98.2-

G

Gas (burned by) Y08.89-

Glass (sharp) X99.0-

Gunshot (wound) – *see* Assault, firearm by type

H

Homicide (attempted) NOS Y09

Hot
- appliances (household) X98.3-
- fluids X98.2-
- other specified objects X98.8-
- unspecified objects X98.9-
- vapors X98.0-
- water (tap) X98.1-

I

Incendiary device X97-

Injury Y09

K

Killed, killing (involving) NOS (*see also* Injury) X58-
- brawl, fight (hand) (fists) (foot) Y04.0-
- cutting, piercing —*see* Assault, cutting or piercing Instrument
- firearm —*see* Discharge, firearm, by type
- knife X99.1-
- steam X98.0-
- toxic gas —*see* Table of Drugs and Chemicals
- vapors Y98.0-

Knife X99.1-

Knocked down (in brawl, fight) Y04.0-

L

Late effect of – *see* X92-Y08 with 7th character S

M

Manslaughter (attempted) Y09-

Murder (attempted) Y09-

P

Perpetrator (person who injured patient) of assault, maltreatment and neglect (by) Y07.9
- boyfriend Y07.03
- brother Y07.410
    - stepbrother V07.435
- coach Y07.53
- Cousin
    - female Y07.491
    - male Y07.490
- daycare provider Y07.519
    - patient in day care center
        - adult care Y07.513
        - childcare Y07.511
    - patient in his/her home
        - adult care Y07.512
        - childcare Y07.510
- family member NEC Y07.499
- father (biological) Y07.11
    - adoptive Y07.13
    - foster Y07.420
    - stepfather Y07.430
- friend of parent (living in home) Y07.59
    - male Y07.432
    - female Y07.434
- girlfriend Y07.04
- healthcare provider Y07.529 – *see also* specific provider
- husband Y07.01
- mental health provider Y07.521
- mother (biological) Y07.12
    - adoptive Y07.14
    - foster Y07.421
    - stepmother Y07.433
- multiple perpetrators Y07.6-
- nonfamily member NOS Y07.59
- nurse Y07.528
- occupational therapist Y07.528
- partner of parent (living in home) Y07.59
    - female Y07.434
    - male Y07.432
- physical therapist Y07.528
- sister Y07.411
    - stepsister Y07.436
- speech therapist Y07.528
- teacher Y07.53
- unspecified perpetrator Y07.9
- wife Y07.02

Accidents, Other – Exposure to, cold to electrical current

NONACCIDENTS, Assault

P (continued)	V
Placing before moving object NEC Y02.8- *see also* Pushing	**Vapors (hot)** X98.0-
motor vehicle Y02.0-	**Violence NOS** Y09
railway vehicle (train) Y02.1-	W
subway train Y02.1-	**Weapon** Y09
Poisoning —*see* categories T36-T65 with 7th character S	blunt object Y00-
Puncture, any part of body —*see* Assault, cutting or piercing instrument	cutting or piercing – *see* Assault, cutting or piercing Instrument
Pushing, pushed	firearm – *see* Assault, discharge, firearm
before moving object NEC Y02.8-	**Wound** (due to) Y09
motor vehicle Y02.0-	blunt object Y00-
railway vehicle (train) Y02.1-	cutting – *see* Assault, cutting or piercing instrument
subway train Y02.1-	gunshot- *see* Assault, discharge, firearm
from high place Y01-	knife X99.1-
R	piercing – *see* Assault, cutting or piercing instrument
Rape (confirmed only) (attempted) T74.2-	puncture – *see* Assault, cutting or piercing instrument
Run over (by) motor vehicle Y03.0 – *see also* Crash	stab – *see* Assault, cutting or piercing instrument
S	
Scald, scalding – *see* Assault, burning	
Scratched by (in fight) Y04.0-	
Sequelae of —*see* X92-Y08 with 7th character S	
Sexual assault (by bodily force) T74.2-	
Sharp object X99.9-	
dagger X99.2-	
glass X99.0-	
knife X99.1-	
object NEC X99.8-	
object NOS X99.9-	
sword X99.2-	
Shooting, shot —*see* Discharge, firearm, by type	
Sodomy (attempted) by force T74.2-	
Specified means NEC Y08.89-	
Stab, any part of body —*see* Assault, cutting or piercing Instrument	
Steam X98.0-	
Strangulation T71-	
Striking against or Struck by	
other person Y04.2-	
sports equipment Y08.09-	
baseball bat Y08.02-	
hockey stick Y08.01-	
other specified equipment V08.9-	
Submersion —*see* Assault, Drowning or submersion	

Note: These codes are for injuries due to assaults not involving a patient who is in the military or law enforcement.

END OF INJURY, DUE TO ASSAULT, HOMICIDE (ATTEMPTED)

CATEGORY – INTENT/CAUSE - NONACCIDENTS
Legal Intervention

B
Blow
by law-enforcing agent, police (on duty) —*see* Legal, intervention, manhandling
blunt object —*see* Legal, intervention, blunt object
bayonet wound in legal intervention —*see* Legal, intervention, sharp object, bayonet
Blunt object
baton
patient was BYSTANDER Y35.312-
patient LAW ENFORCEMENT PERSONNEL Y35.311-
patient was SUSPECT Y35.313-
unspecified person Y35.319-
other specified blunt object
patient was BYSTANDER Y35.392-
patient LAW ENFORCEMENT PERSONNEL Y35.391-
patient was SUSPECT Y35.393-
unspecified person Y35.399-
unspecified blunt object
patient was BYSTANDER Y35.302-
patient LAW ENFORCEMENT PERSONNEL Y35.301-
patient was SUSPECT Y35.303-
unspecified person Y35.309-
wooden post or plank (stave) (truncheon)
patient was BYSTANDER Y35.392-
patient LAW ENFORCEMENT PERSONNEL Y35.391-
patient was SUSPECT Y35.393-
unspecified person Y35.399-
Bomb —*see* Legal intervention, explosive

C
Cut, cutting (any part of body) – *see* Legal intervention, sharp Object

D
Discharge (firearms)
handgun
patient was BYSTANDER Y35.022-
patient LAW ENFORCEMENT PERSONNEL Y35.021-
patient was SUSPECT Y35.023-
unspecified person Y35.029-
machine gun
patient was BYSTANDER Y35.012-
patient LAW ENFORCEMENT PERSONNEL Y35.011-
patient was SUSPECT Y35.013-
unspecified person Y35.019-

D (continued)
Discharge (firearms) (continued)
rifle pellet
patient was BYSTANDER Y35.032-
patient LAW ENFORCEMENT PERSONNEL Y35.031-
patient was SUSPECT Y35.033-
unspecified person Y35.039-
rubber bullet
patient was BYSTANDER Y35.042-
patient LAW ENFORCEMENT PERSONNEL Y35.041-
patient was SUSPECT Y35.043-
unspecified person Y35.049-
shotgun – *see* Legal intervention, firearm, specified NEC
specified NEC
patient was BYSTANDER Y35.092-
patient LAW ENFORCEMENT PERSONNEL Y35.091-
patient was SUSPECT Y35.093-
unspecified person Y35.0939-
unspecified firearm
patient was BYSTANDER Y35.002-
patient LAW ENFORCEMENT PERSONNEL Y35.001-
patient was SUSPECT Y35.003-
unspecified person Y35.009-
Dragged (manhandled)
patient was BYSTANDER Y35.812-
patient LAW ENFORCEMENT PERSONNEL Y35.811-
patient was SUSPECT Y35.813-
unspecified person Y35.819-
Dynamite – *see* Explosives, dynamite

Note: These codes are for injuries involving a patient who is law enforcement personnel, a suspect or a bystander during a legal intervention.

NONACCIDENTS, Legal Intervention

E
Electroshock device – *see* Taser, Stun gun
Explosives
dynamite
patient was BYSTANDER Y35.112-
patient LAW ENFORCEMENT PERSONNEL Y35.111-
patient was SUSPECT Y35.113-
unspecified person Y35.119-
explosive shell – *see* Shell
grenade
patient was BYSTANDER Y35.192-
patient LAW ENFORCEMENT PERSONNEL Y35.191-
patient was SUSPECT Y35.193-
unspecified person Y35.199-
mortar bomb
patient was BYSTANDER Y35.192-
patient LAW ENFORCEMENT PERSONNEL Y35.191-
patient was SUSPECT Y35.193-
unspecified person Y35.199-
shell (explosive)
patient was BYSTANDER Y35.122-
patient LAW ENFORCEMENT PERSONNEL Y35.121-
patient was SUSPECT Y35.123-
unspecified person Y35.129-
specified NEC
patient was BYSTANDER Y35.192-
patient LAW ENFORCEMENT PERSONNEL Y35.191-
patient was SUSPECT Y35.193-
unspecified person Y35.199-
unspecified explosive NOS
patient was BYSTANDER Y35.102-
patient LAW ENFORCEMENT PERSONNEL Y35.101-
patient was SUSPECT Y35.103-
unspecified person Y35.109-

G
Gas (asphyxiation) (poisoning) (injuring)
specified NEC
patient was BYSTANDER Y35.292-
patient LAW ENFORCEMENT PERSONNEL Y35.291-
patient was SUSPECT Y35.293-
unspecified person Y35.299-
tear gas
patient was BYSTANDER Y35.212-
patient LAW ENFORCEMENT PERSONNEL Y35.211-
patient was SUSPECT Y35.213-
unspecified person Y35.219-
unspecified gas
patient was BYSTANDER Y35.202-
patient LAW ENFORCEMENT PERSONNEL Y35.201-
patient was SUSPECT Y35.203-
unspecified person Y35.209-

K
Kicked (manhandled)
patient was BYSTANDER Y35.812-
patient LAW ENFORCEMENT PERSONNEL Y35.811-
patient was SUSPECT Y35.813-
unspecified person Y35.819-

L
Late effect (of legal intervention)-*see* Y35.9 with 7th character S

M
Manhandled (roughly dragged, kicked or pushed)
patient was BYSTANDER Y35.812-
patient LAW ENFORCEMENT PERSONNEL Y35.811-
patient was SUSPECT Y35.813-
unspecified person Y35.819-

P
Poisoning (by) – *see also* Table of Drugs and Chemicals
gas – *see* Legal intervention, gas
Pushed (manhandled)
patient was BYSTANDER Y35.812-
patient LAW ENFORCEMENT PERSONNEL Y35.811-
patient was SUSPECT Y35.813-
unspecified person Y35.819-

List intent/cause codes before other External Cause codes.
Use more than one code if needed to completely explain
The circumstances. **Use these codes throughout treatment with applicable 7th character.**

Nonaccidents, Legal Intervention, Scratched by to Unspecified injury

NONACCIDENTS, Legal Intervention

S
Scratched by (injuring patient)
patient was BYSTANDER Y35.892-
patient LAW ENFORCEMENT Y35.891-
patient was SUSPECT Y35.893-
unspecified person Y35.899-
Sequelae (of legal intervention) - see Y35.9 with 7th character S
Sharp objects
bayonet
patient was BYSTANDER Y35.412-
patient LAW ENFORCEMENT PERSONNEL Y35.411-
patient was SUSPECT Y35.413
unspecified person Y35.419-
specified sharp object NEC
patient was BYSTANDER Y35.492-
patient LAW ENFORCEMENT PERSONNEL Y35.491-
patient was SUSPECT Y35.493-
unspecified person Y35.499-
unspecified sharp object
patient was BYSTANDER Y35.402-
patient LAW ENFORCEMENT PERSONNEL Y35.401-
patient was SUSPECT Y35.403-
unspecified person Y35.409-
Specified means of injury NEC
patient was BYSTANDER Y35.892-
patient LAW ENFORCEMENT PERSONNEL Y35.891-
patient was SUSPECT Y35.893-
unspecified person Y35.899-
Stabbing – see Legal intervention, sharp object
Stave – see Legal, intervention, blunt object, stave
Struck by (injuring patient)
other person(s)
patient was BYSTANDER Y35.812-
patient LAW ENFORCEMENT PERSONNEL Y35.811-
patient was SUSPECT Y35.813-
unspecified person Y35.819-
police (on duty) —see Legal, intervention, manhandling
with blunt object —see Legal, intervention, blunt object
Stun gun
patient was BYSTANDER Y35.832-
patient LAW ENFORCEMENT PERSONNEL Y35.831-
patient was SUSPECT Y35.833-
unspecified person Y35.839-

T
Taser
patient was BYSTANDER Y35.832-
patient LAW ENFORCEMENT PERSONNEL Y35.831-
patient was SUSPECT Y35.833-
unspecified person Y35.839-
Tear gas – see Legal intervention, gas, tear gas
Truncheon – see Legal, intervention, blunt object, stave

U
Unspecified injury
patient was BYSTANDER Y35.92-
patient LAW ENFORCEMENT PERSONNEL Y35.91-
patient was SUSPECT Y35.93-
unspecified person Y35.99-

Note: These codes are for injuries involving a patient who is law enforcement personnel, a suspect or a bystander during a legal intervention.

END OF INJURY, DUE TO LEGAL INTERVENTIONS

CATEGORY – INTENT/CAUSE - NONACCIDENTS
Self-Harm

A
Appliance (hot) X77.3-
Aircraft (crashing) X83.0-
Asphyxia, asphyxiation X83.8-
B
Blunt object X79-
Bomb – *see* Explosion
Burn, burned, burning (from) (hot)
appliance (electrical) (household) X77.3-
caustic or corrosive substance (swallowed) – *see* Table of Drugs and Chemicals
fluids (other) X77.2-
hotplate X77.3-
iron (hot) X77.3-
other specified hot object NEC X77.8-
steam X77.0-
tap water X77.1-
unspecified object NOS X77.9-
vapors X77.0-
C
Caustic or corrosive substance (swallowed) – *see* Table of Drugs and Chemicals
Cold, extreme X83.2-
Collision of motor vehicle (with)
motor vehicle (two vehicles collided) X82.0-
other specified collision X82.8-
railway vehicle (train) X82.1-
tree X82.2-
Contact with – *see also* Cut, Cutting or piercing or Burn
cooker (hot) X77.3-
fluids (hot) X77.2-
household appliance X77.3-
lawnmower (powered) (ridden) X83.1-
liquid (boiling) (hot) X77.2-
other specified hot object NEC X77.8-
tap water X77.1-
Crash – *see also* Collision of motor vehicle
aircraft (in transit) (powered) X83.0-

C (continued)
Cut (any part of body) X78.9-
Cutting or piercing instrument (using sharp object) X78.9-
dagger X78.2-
glass X78.0-
knife X78.1-
other specified sharp object X78.8-
sword X78.2-
unspecified sharp object X78.9-
D
Discharge (firearm) X74.9-
air gun X74.01-
BB gun X74.01-
flare X74.8-
gas-operated gun NEC X74.09-
handgun (pistol) (revolver) X72-
hunting rifle X73.1-
large firearm NEC X73.8-
large firearm NOS X73.9-
machine gun X73.2-
paintball gun X74.02-
pellet gun X74.01-
pistol X72-
revolver X72-
rifle (hunting) X73.1-
shotgun X73.0-
other (large) specified firearm X73.9-
spring-operated gun NEC X74.09-
unspecified firearm X74.9-
Very pistol X74.8-
Drowning or submersion (patient in) (involving) X71.9-
bathtub X71.0-
natural water (lake) (open sea) (river) (stream) (pond) X71.3-
specified place NEC X71.8-
swimming pool
in pool X71.1-
following fall or jump into pool X71.2-
other specified drowning or submersion X71.8-
unspecified circumstances X71.9-

List intent/cause codes before other External Cause codes. Use more than one code if needed to completely explain the circumstances. **Use these codes throughout treatment with applicable 7th character.**

Nonaccidents, Self-harm, Electrocution to Wound NEC

NONACCIDENTS, Self-Harm

E
Electrocution X83.1-
Explosion (any) (bomb) (grenade) X75-
Exposure (to)
- cold (excessive) (extreme) (natural) (place) X83.2-
- electric current X83.1-
- fire, flames X76-
- taser X83.8-

F
Fall, falling X80 – *see* Jumped
Fire, flames X76-
Firearms – *see* Discharge, firearms
Fluids (hot) – *see* Burn

G
Grenade – *see* Explosion

H
Hanging X83.8-
Hot – *see* Burning, hot object

J
Jumped, jumping
- before (in front of) moving object X81.8-
  - motor vehicle X81.0-
  - other moving object X81.8-
  - railway vehicle (train) X81.1-
    - subway train X81.1-
- from high place X80-
- into natural water (resulting in drowning or submersion) X71.3-
- into swimming pool (resulting in drowning or submersion) X71.2-

L
Late effect of attempted self-harm — *see* X71-X83 with 7th character S
Lying before vehicle – *see* Jumped

M
Motor vehicle – *see* Collision or Lying before vehicle

O
Object – *see* Blunt object or Cutting or piercing object
Other specified means of self-harm X83.8-

P
Piercing object – *see* Cutting or piercing object
Poisoning —*see* Table of Drugs and Chemicals
Puncture (any part of body) —*see* Suicide, cutting or piercing instrument

R
Running before moving object X81.8- *see also* Jumped
- motor vehicle X81.0-

S
Scald —*see* Suicide, burning, hot object
Sequelae of attempted self-harm — *see* X71-X83 with 7th character S
Sharp object (any) —*see* Suicide, cutting or piercing instrument
Shooting —*see* Suicide, discharge (firearm)
Smoke X76-
Specified means NEC X83.8-
Stab (any part of body) —*see* Suicide, cutting or piercing instrument
Steam, hot vapors X77.0-
Strangulation X83.8-
Submersion —*see* Suicide, Drowning or submersion
Suffocation X83.8-
Swimming pool – *see* Drowning or submersion, Jumped

T
Toxic gas —*see* Table of Drugs and Chemicals

V
Vapors X77.0-

W
Water (hot) (tap) X77.1-
Wound NEC X83.8-

These codes are for injuries involving a patient who intentionally injures him/herself, including attempting suicide.

END OF INJURY, DUE TO SUICIDE (SELF-HARM)

CATEGORY – INTENT/CAUSE – NONACCIDENTS
Terrorism

A	
Aircraft destruction – *see* Destruction of aircraft	
Aerial bomb – *see* Explosion, bomb	
Anthrax – *see* Biological weapons	
Antipersonnel bomb – *see* Explosion, bomb	
Artillery shell – *see* Explosion, other	
B	
Biological weapons Y38.6X-	
	patient is CIVILIAN V38.6X2-
	patient is PUBLIC SAFETY OFFICIAL V38.6X1-
	patient is TERRORIST V38.6X3-
Blast (fragments) Y38.20- *See also* Explosion or Fragments	
	patient is CIVILIAN V38.2X2-
	patient is PUBLIC SAFETY OFFICIAL V38.2X1-
	patient is TERRORIST V38.2X3-
Bomb Y38.2X- - *see* Explosion, Fragments, Fire or Suicide bomber	
Breech block – *see* Explosion, other	
Burn – *see* Fire	
	aircraft – *see* Destruction of aircraft
C	
Cannon block – *see* Explosion, other	
Chemical weapons Y38.7X-	
	patient is CIVILIAN Y38.7X2-
	patient is PUBLIC SAFETY OFFICIAL Y38.7X1-
	patient is TERRORIST Y38.7X3-
Cholera – *see* Biological weapons	
Conflagration – *see* Fire	
Cut, cutting - see Piercing or stabbing instrument	
D	
Depth-charge – *see* Explosion, marine weapon	
Destruction of aircraft Y38.1-	
	patient is CIVILIAN Y38.1X2-
	patient is PUBLIC SAFETY OFFICIAL Y38.1X1-
	patient is TERRORIST Y38.1X3-
Dirty bomb – *see* Explosion, bomb, other	
Discharge (firearm) (any type of firearm) Y38.4X-	
	patient is CIVILIAN Y38.4X2-
	patient is PUBLIC SAFETY OFFICIAL Y38.4X1-
	patient is TERRORIST Y38.4X3-
Drowning or submersion Y38.89-	
	patient is CIVILIAN Y38.892-
	patient is PUBLIC SAFETY OFFICIAL Y38.891-
	patient is TERRORIST Y38.893-

E	
Explosion (of) Y38.2X- - *see also* Bomb or Fragments	
	aircraft – *see* Destruction, aircraft
	bomb (includes aerial, antipersonnel, dirty bomb, gasoline bomb, land mine, mortar) – *see also* Suicide Bomber
	patient is CIVILIAN Y38.2X2-
	patient is PUBLIC SAFETY OFFICIAL Y38.2X1-
	patient is TERRORIST Y38.2X3-
	marine weapon (includes depth-charge, marine mine, sea-based artillery shell, torpedo, underwater blast) Y38.0X-
	patient is CIVILIAN Y38.0X2-
	patient is PUBLIC SAFETY OFFICIAL Y38.0X1-
	patient is TERRORIST Y38.0X3-
	other explosions (includes artillery shell, breech block, cannon block, depth-charge, grenade, guided missile, munitions, rocket, mine NOS) Y38.2X-
	patient is CIVILIAN Y38.2X2-
	patient is PUBLIC SAFETY OFFICIAL Y38.2X1-
	patient is TERRORIST Y38.2X3-
F	
Fire Y38.3X- (includes petrol bomb, conflagration, hot substance)	
	patient is CIVILIAN Y38.3X2-
	patient is PUBLIC SAFETY OFFICIAL Y38.3X1-
	patient is TERRORIST Y38.3X3-
Firearms – *see* Discharge (firearms)	
Fragments (includes fragments of artillery shell, bomb, grenade, guided missile, land mine, rocket, shell, shrapnel) Y38.2X- - *see also* Explosion	
	patient is CIVILIAN Y38.2X2-
	patient is PUBLIC SAFETY OFFICIAL Y38.2X1-
	patient is TERRORIST Y38.2X3-
G	
Gas – *see* Chemical weapons	
Gasoline bomb – *see* Explosion, bomb or Fire	
Grenade – *see* Explosion, other	
Guided missile – *see* Explosion, other	

These codes are for injuries involving a patient who is a terrorist, public safety official (law enforcement official, firefighter, chaplain, member of rescue squad or ambulance crew), or a bystander during a terrorist event.

Terrorism must be confirmed as such by the FBI. If not confirmed by the FBI (suspected terrorism), use assault codes.

Nonaccidents, Terrorism, Hot substance to Weapons

NONACCIDENTS, Terrorism

H
Hot substances (any) Y38.3X-
patient is CIVILIAN Y38.3X2-
patient is PUBLIC SAFETY OFFICER Y38.3X1-
patient is TERRORIST Y38.3X3-
Hydrogen cyanide – *see* Chemical weapons

L
Land mine – *see* Explosion, bomb

M
Marine mine – *see* Explosion, marine weapon
Mine NOS – *see* Explosion
Mortar bomb – *see* Explosion, bomb
Munitions – *see* Explosion, other

N
Nuclear weapon (effects of) Y38.5X-
patient is CIVILIAN Y38.5X2-
patient is PUBLIC SAFETY OFFICIAL Y38.5X1-
patient is TERRORIST Y38.5X3-

O
Other specified means Y38.891-
patient is CIVILIAN Y38.892-
patient is PUBLIC SAFETY OFFICIAL Y38.891-
patient is TERRORIST Y38.893-

P
Petrol bomb – *see* Fire
Piercing (cutting) or stabbing object Y38.89-
patient is CIVILIAN Y38.892-
patient is PUBLIC SAFETY OFFICIAL Y38.891-
patient is TERRORIST Y38.893-
Phosgene – *see* Chemical weapons

R
Rocket – *see* Explosion, other

S
Sarin – *see* Chemical weapons
Sea-based artillery shell – *see* Explosion, marine weapon
Secondary effects of terrorism (injury occurring after initial attack) Y38.9-
patient is CIVILIAN Y38.9X2-
patient is PUBLIC SAFETY OFFICIAL Y38.9X1-
Shot down (aircraft) – *see* Destruction, aircraft
Shrapnel NOS - *see* Fragments
Smallpox – *see* Biological weapons
Stabbing – *see* Piercing or stabbing instrument
Submersion – *see* Drowning or submersion
Suicide bomber Y38.81-
patient is CIVILIAN Y38.812-
patient is PUBLIC SAFETY OFFICIAL Y38.811-

T
Torpedo – *see* Explosion, marine weapon

U
Underwater blast – *see* Explosion, marine weapon
Unspecified means Y38.80-

W
Weapons
biological – *see* Biological weapons
bombs – *see* Explosion
chemical – *see* Chemical weapons
nuclear – *see* Nuclear weapons
specified NEC – *see* Other specified means
weapon of mass destruction [WMD] – *see* Explosion

List terrorism codes before other intent/cause codes. Use more than one code if needed to completely explain the circumstances. **Use these codes throughout treatment with applicable 7th Character.**

END OF INJURY, DUE TO TERRORISM

CATEGORY – INTENT/CAUSE – NONACCIDENTS
Undetermined

B
Bayonet wound Y28.8-
Blunt object Y29-
Burn, burned, burning
household appliance Y27.3
internal, from swallowed caustic, corrosive liquid, substance - see Table of Drugs and Chemicals

C
Contact with (hot)
dagger Y28.2-
fluids NEC Y27.2-
glass (sharp) (broken) Y28.0-
household appliance Y27.3-
knife Y28.1-
liquid NEC Y27.2-
steam Y27.0-
sword Y28.2-
unspecified object (hot) Y27.9-
vapors Y27.0-
water (in bathtub) (on stove) Y27.1-
Crashing of motor vehicle Y32-

D
Discharge (firearm) Y24.9-
air gun Y24.0-
BB gun Y24.0-
flare gun Y24.8-
gas-operated gun NEC Y24.8-
handgun (pistol) (revolver) Y22-
hunting rifle Y23.1-
machine gun Y23.3-
military firearm Y23.2-
other large firearm Y23.8-
paintball gun Y24.8-
pellet gun Y24.0-
rifle (hunting) Y23.1-
shotgun Y23.0-
unspecified firearm Y23.9-
Very pistol Y24.8-

D (continued)
Drowning or submersion (patient in) (involving) Y21.9-
bathtub
after fall into bathtub Y21.1-
while in bathtub Y21.0-
natural water (lake) (open sea) (river) (stream) (pond) Y21.4-
specified place NEC Y21.8-
swimming pool
after fall into pool Y21.3-
while in swimming pool Y21.2-
unspecified place Y21.9-

E
Explosion Y25-

F
Fall, falling
high place NEC Y30-
falling, lying or running before moving object Y31-
Fire or flame Y26-
Firearm discharge – see Discharge (firearm)
Firework (s) – Y25-

H
Hot object – see Contact with (hot) or Scald

These codes are used only when the physician specifically documents the intent as undetermined (cannot be clinically determined).

Nonaccidents, Undetermined, Jumped to Swimming pool

NONACCIDENTS, Undetermined

J
Jumped, jumping
before moving object NEC Y31-
from high place NEC Y30-
K
Killed, killing NOS - *see also* Injury Y33-
L
Lying before train, vehicle or other moving object Y31-
M
Motor vehicle crash (collision) Y32-
P
Push, fall or jump from high place Y30-
R
Running, falling or lying before moving object Y31-

S
Scald, scalding
hot tap water Y27.2-
household appliance Y27.3-
liquid (boiling) (hot) NEC Y27.2-
steam Y27.0-
unspecified object Y28.9-
vapors (hot) Y27.0-
Sharp object Y28.9-
dagger Y28.2-
glass Y28.0-
knife Y28.1-
specified sharp object NEC Y28.8-
sword Y28.2-
unspecified sharp object Y28.9-
Slashed wrists —*see* Contact with or Sharp object
Smoke Y26-
Specified event NEC Y33-
Struck by
blunt object Y29-
other person (s) with blunt object Y29-
Submersion – *see* Drowning or submersion
Swimming pool – *see* Drowning or submersion

List intent/cause codes before other External Cause codes. Use more than one code if needed to completely explain the circumstances. **Use these codes throughout treatment with applicable 7th character.**

END OF INJURY, UNDETERMINED INTENT

CATEGORY – INTENT/CAUSE - MILITARY
Military Operations

A
Air blast – see Explosion, Fragments
Aircraft destruction – see Destruction, aircraft
Airway restriction – see Restriction of airway
Anthrax – see Biological weapons
Asphyxiation —see Restriction of airways

B
Biological weapons Y37.6X-
patient is CIVILIAN Y37.6X1-
patient is MILITARY PERSONNEL Y37.6X0-
Blast (fragments) – see Fragments
Blunt object Y37.45-
patient is CIVILIAN Y37.451-
patient is MILITARY PERSONNEL Y37.450-
Bomb Y37.20- see also Explosion
aerial bomb Y37.21-
patient is CIVILIAN Y37.211-
patient is MILITARY PERSONNEL Y37.221-
dirty Y37.50-
patient is CIVILIAN Y37.501-
patient is MILITARY PERSONNEL Y37.500-
gasoline (petrol) Y37.31-
patient is CIVILIAN Y37.311-
patient is MILITARY PERSONNEL Y37.310-
incendiary bomb Y37.31- - see also Incendiary bullet
patient is CIVILIAN Y37.311-
patient is MILITARY PERSONNEL Y37.310-
unspecified bomb Y37.20-
patient is CIVILIAN Y37.201-
patient is MILITARY PERSONNEL Y37.200-
Bullet
incendiary Y37.32-
patient is CIVILIAN Y37.431-
patient is MILITARY PERSONNEL Y37.430-
rubber Y37.41-
patient is CIVILIAN Y37.341-
patient is MILITARY PERSONNEL Y37.410-

C
Chemical weapons Y37.7X-
patient is CIVILIAN Y37.7X1-
patient is MILITARY PERSONNEL Y37.7X0-
Choking – see Restriction of airway
Cholera – see Biological weapons
Conflagration – see Fire

These codes are used for injuries involving a patient who is either in the military or a civilian in a military setting. Injury occurred during peacetime, either or military property or during routine military exercises and operations. See also War operations.

C (continued)
Combat
hand to hand (unarmed) combat Y37.44-
patient is CIVILIAN Y37.441-
patient is MILITARY PERSONNEL Y37.440-
using blunt or piercing object Y37.45-
patient is CIVILIAN Y37.451-
patient is MILITARY PERSONNEL Y37.450-
Conventional warfare NEC Y37.49-
patient is CIVILIAN V37.491-
patient is MILITARY PERSONNEL V37.490-
Cutting object – see Piercing object

D
Depth-charge – see Explosion
Destruction of aircraft (due to) Y37.10-
collision with other aircraft Y37.12-
patient is CIVILIAN Y37.121-
patient is MILITARY PERSONNEL Y37.120-
detonation (accidental) of onboard munitions and explosives Y37.14- see also Detonation
patient is CIVILIAN Y37.141-
patient is MILITARY PERSONNEL Y37.140-
enemy fire or explosives Y37.11-
patient is CIVILIAN Y37.111-
patient is MILITARY PERSONNEL Y37.110-
fire onboard aircraft Y37.13-
patient is CIVILIAN Y37.131-
patient is MILITARY PERSONNEL Y37.130-
specified destruction of aircraft NEC Y37.19-
patient is CIVILIAN Y37.191-
patient is MILITARY PERSONNEL Y37.190-
unspecified cause, destruction of aircraft Y37.10-
patient is CIVILIAN Y37.101-
patient is MILITARY PERSONNEL Y37.100-
Detonation (accidental) of – see also Explosion or Fragments
with destruction of aircraft Y37.14-
patient is CIVILIAN Y37.141-
patient is MILITARY PERSONNEL Y37.140-
onboard marine weapons (accidental) Y37.05-
patient is CIVILIAN Y37.051-
patient is MILITARY PERSONNEL Y37.050-
own munitions or munitions launch device (accidental) Y37.24-
patient is CIVILIAN Y37.241-
patient is MILITARY PERSONNEL Y37.240-
Dirty bomb – see Bomb

Military, Military Operations, Discharge to Land mine

MILITARY, Military Operations

D (continued)
Discharge (firearm) (any type) Y37.43- *see also* Bullet
other firearms Y37.43-
patient is CIVILIAN Y37.431-
patient is MILITARY PERSONNEL Y37.430-
pellets Y37.42-
patient is CIVILIAN Y37.421-
patient is MILITARY PERSONNEL Y37.420-
rubber bullets Y37.41-
patient is CIVILIAN Y37.4-
patient is MIITARY PERSONNEL Y37.420-
E
Explosion (of) Y37.20- - *see also* Bomb, Detonation, Fragments
artillery shell (sea based) V37.03-
patient is CIVILIAN V37.031-
patient is MILITARY PERSONNEL Y37.030-
depth-charge Y37.01-
patient is CIVILIAN Y37.011-
patient is MILITARY PERSONNEL Y37.010-
grenade Y37.29-
patient is CIVILIAN Y37.291-
patient is MILITARY PERSONNEL Y37.290-
guided missile Y37.22-
patient is CIVILIAN Y37.221-
patient is MILITARY PERSONNEL Y37.220-
improvised explosive device [IED] (person-borne) (road-side) (vehicle-borne) Y37.23-
patient is CIVILIAN Y37.231-
patient is MILITARY PERSONNEL Y37.230-
land mine Y37.29-
patient is CIVILIAN Y37.291-
patient is MILITARY PERSONNEL Y37.290-
marine mine (at sea) (in harbor) Y37.02-
patient is CIVILIAN Y37.021-
patient is MILITARY PERSONNEL Y37.020-
marine weapon Y37.00-
accidental detonation of onboard marine weapon
patient is CIVILIAN Y37.051-
patient is MILITARY PERSONNEL Y37.050-
other specified – *see also* specific weapon Y37.09-
patient is CIVILIAN Y37.091-
patient is MILITARY PERSONNEL Y37.090-
unspecified marine weapon Y37.0-
patient is CIVILIAN Y37.001-
patient is MILITARY PERSONNEL Y37.000-
munitions or munitions launch device Y37.24-
patient is CIVILIAN Y37.241-
patient is MILITARY PERSONNEL Y37.240-

F
Fire Y37.30- *see also* Flamethrower
specified fire NEC Y37.39-
patient is CIVILIAN Y37.391-
patient is MILITARY PERSONNEL Y37.390-
unspecified fire NOS Y37.30-
patient is CIVILIAN Y37.301-
patient is MILITARY PERSONNEL Y37.300-
Firearms – *see* Discharge (firearms)
Flamethrower Y37.33-
patient is CIVILIAN Y37.331-
patient is MILITARY PERSONNEL Y37.330-
Fragments (from) (of)
improvised explosive device [IED] (person-borne) (road-side) (vehicle-borne) Y37.26-
patient is CIVILIAN Y37.261-
patient is MILITARY PERSONNEL Y37.260-
munitions Y37.25-
patient is CIVILIAN Y37.251-
patient is MILITARY PERSONNEL Y37.250-
specified NEC Y37.29-
patient is CIVILIAN Y37.291-
patient is MILITARY PERSONNEL Y37.290-
weapons Y37.27-
patient is CIVILIAN Y37.271-
patient is MILITARY PERSONNEL Y37.270-
Friendly fire Y37.92-
G
Gas – *see* Chemical weapons
Gasoline bomb – *see* Bomb
Grenade – *see* Explosion
Guided missile – *see* Explosion
H
Hand to hand (unarmed) combat Y37.44-
patient is CIVILIAN Y37.441-
patient is MILITARY PERSONNEL Y37.440-
Hot substances Y37.30-
specified substance NEC Y37.30-
patient is CIVILIAN Y37.390-
patient is MILITARY PERSONNEL Y37.391-
unspecified substance NOS Y37.30-
patient is CIVILIAN Y37.301-
patient is MILITARY PERSONNEL Y37.300-
Hydrogen cyanide – *see* Chemical weapons
I
Incendiary bullet – *see* Bullet
L
Land mine – *see* Explosion, bomb

MILITARY, Military Operations

M		R	
Marine mine – *see* Explosion, marine weapon		**Restriction of air** (airway) (choking) Y37.4-	
Mine NOS – *see* Explosion			intentional (on purpose) Y37.46-
Mortar bomb – *see* Bomb, unspecified			patient is CIVILIAN Y37.461-
Munitions – *see* Explosion			patient is MILITARY PERSONNEL Y37.460-
N			unintentional (accidental) Y37.47-
Nuclear weapon (effects of) Y37.50-			patient is CIVILIAN Y37.471-
	acute radiation exposure Y37.54- see Nuclear radiation		patient is MILITARY PERSONNEL Y37.470-
	direct blast Y37.51-	S	
	patient is CIVILIAN Y37.511-	**Sarin** – *see* Chemical weapons	
	patient is MILITARY PERSONNEL Y37.510-	**Shot down (aircraft)** – *see* Destruction, aircraft	
	direct heat - see Nuclear weapon, thermal radiation	**Shrapnel NOS** Y37.29- *see also* Fragments	
	fallout exposure – see Nuclear weapon, nuclear radiation		patient is CIVILIAN Y37.291-
	fireball Y37.53-		patient is MILITARY PERSONNEL Y37.290-
	patient is CIVILIAN Y37.531-	**Smallpox** – *see* Biological weapons	
	patient is MILITARY PERSONNEL Y37.530-	**Stabbing** – *see* Piercing object	
	indirect blast Y37.52-	**Suffocation** —*see* Restriction of airways	
	patient is CIVILIAN Y37.521-	T	
	patient is MILITARY PERSONNEL Y37.520-	**Torpedo** – *see* Explosion, marine weapon	
	nuclear radiation Y37.54-	U	
	patient is CIVILIAN Y37.541-	**Unconventional warfare NEC** Y37.7X- *see also* Chemical and Biological warfare	
	patient is MILITARY PERSONNEL Y37.540-		patient is CIVILIAN Y37.7X1-
	secondary effects Y37.54-		patient is MILITARY PERSONNEL Y37.7X0-
	patient is CIVILIAN Y37.541-	**Underwater blast NOS** Y37.00-	
	patient is MILITARY PERSONNEL Y37.540-		patient is CIVILIAN Y37.001-
	specified effects Y37.59-		patient is MILITARY PERSONNEL Y37.000-
	patient is CIVILIAN Y37.591-	**Unspecified means** Y37.90-	
	patient is MILITARY PERSONNEL Y37.590-	W	
	thermal radiation Y37.53-	**Warfare**	
	patient is CIVILIAN Y37.531-		conventional NEC Y37.49-
	patient is MILITARY PERSONNEL Y37.530-		patient is CIVILIAN Y37.490-
	unspecified effects Y37.50-		patient is MILITARY PERSONNEL Y37.491-
	patient is CIVILIAN Y37.351-		unconventional NEC Y37.7X-
	patient is MILITARY PERSONNEL Y37.450-		patient is CIVILIAN Y37.590-
O			patient is MILITARY PERSONNEL Y37.591-
Object – *see* Blunt or Piercing		**Weapons**	
Other specified means V37.90-			biological – see Biological weapons
P			chemical – see Chemical weapons
Petrol bomb – *see* Fire			nuclear – see Nuclear weapons (effects of)
Phosgene – *see* Chemical weapons			specified NEC Y37.59-
Piercing (cutting) object Y37.45-			weapon of mass destruction [WMD] Y37.9-
	patient is CIVILIAN Y37.451-		
	patient is MILITARY PERSONNEL Y37.450-		

These codes are used for injuries involving a patient who is either in the military or a civilian in a military setting. Injury occurred during peacetime, either on military property or during routine military exercises and operations. See also War operations.

List intent/cause codes before other External Cause codes. Use more than one code if needed to completely explain the circumstances. **Use these codes throughout treatment with applicable 7th character.**

END OF INJURY, DURING MILITARY OPERATIONS

CATEGORY – INTENT/CAUSE – MILITARY
War Operations

A
- **Air blast** – see Explosion, Fragments
- **Aircraft destruction** – see Destruction, aircraft
- **Airway restriction** – see Restriction of airway
- **Anthrax** – see Biological weapons
- **Asphyxiation** —see Restriction of airways

B
- **Biological weapons** Y36.6X-
  - patient is CIVILIAN Y36.6X1-
  - patient is MILITARY PERSONNEL Y36.6X0-
- **Blast (fragments)** – see Fragments
- **Blunt object** Y36.45-
  - patient is CIVILIAN Y36.451-
  - patient is MILITARY PERSONNEL Y36.450-
- **Bomb** – see also Explosion
  - aerial bomb Y36.21-
    - patient is CIVILIAN Y36.211-
    - patient is MILITARY PERSONNEL Y36.210-
  - dirty Y36.50-
    - patient is CIVILIAN Y36.501-
    - patient is MILITARY PERSONNEL Y36.500-
  - exploding after cessation of hostilities Y36.8-
    - patient is CIVILIAN Y36.811-
    - patient is MILITARY PERSONNEL Y36.810-
  - gasoline (petrol) Y36.31-
    - patient is CIVILIAN Y36.311-
    - patient is MILITARY PERSONNEL Y36.310-
  - incendiary bomb Y36.31- - see also Incendiary bullet
    - patient is CIVILIAN Y36.311-
    - patient is MILITARY PERSONNEL Y36.310-
  - unspecified bomb Y36.20-
    - patient is CIVILIAN Y36.201-
    - patient is MILITARY PERSONNEL Y36.200-
- **Bullet**
  - incendiary Y36.32-
    - patient is CIVILIAN Y36.321-
    - patient is MILITARY PERSONNEL Y36.320-
  - rubber Y36.41-
    - patient is CIVILIAN Y36.411-
    - patient is MILITARY PERSONNEL Y36.410-

C
- **Chemical weapons** Y36.7X-
  - patient is CIVILIAN Y36.7X1-
  - patient is MILITARY PERSONNEL Y36.7X0-
- **Choking** – see Restriction of airway

C (continued)
- **Combat**
  - hand to hand (unarmed) combat Y36.44-
    - patient is CIVILIAN Y36.3441-
    - patient is MILITARY PERSONNEL Y36.440-
  - using blunt or piercing object Y36.45-
    - patient is CIVILIAN Y36.451-
    - patient is MILITARY PERSONNEL Y36.450-
- **Conflagration** – see Fire
- **Conventional warfare NEC** Y36.49-
  - patient is CIVILIAN Y36.491-
  - patient is MILITARY PERSONNEL Y36.490-
- **Cutting object** – see Piercing object

D
- **Depth-charge** – see Explosion
- **Destruction of aircraft (due to)** Y36.10-
  - collision with other aircraft Y36.12-
    - patient is CIVILIAN Y36.121-
    - patient is MILITARY PERSONNEL Y36.120-
  - detonation (accidental) of onboard munitions and explosives Y36.14- see also Detonation
    - patient is CIVILIAN Y36.141-
    - patient is MILITARY PERSONNEL Y36.140-
  - enemy fire or explosives Y36.11-
    - patient is CIVILIAN Y36.111-
    - patient is MILITARY PERSONNEL Y36.110-
  - fire onboard aircraft Y36.13-
    - patient is CIVILIAN Y36.131-
    - patient is MILITARY PERSONNEL Y36.130-
  - specified destruction of aircraft NEC Y36.19-
    - patient is CIVILIAN Y36.191-
    - patient is MILITARY PERSONNEL Y36.190-
  - unspecified cause Y36.10-
    - patient is CIVILIAN Y36.101-
    - patient is MILITARY PERSONNEL Y36.100-
- **Detonation (accidental) of** – see also Explosion or Fragments
  - with destruction of aircraft Y36.14-
    - patient is CIVILIAN Y36.141-
    - patient is MILITARY PERSONNEL Y36.140-
  - onboard marine weapons (accidental) Y36.05-
    - patient is CIVILIAN Y36.051-
    - patient is MILITARY PERSONNEL Y36.050-
  - own munitions or munitions launch device Y36.24-
    - patient is CIVILIAN Y36.241-
    - patient is MILITARY PERSONNEL Y36.240-
- **Dirty bomb** - see Bomb

MILITARY, War Operations

D (continued)
Discharge (firearm) (any type) Y36.43- *see also* Bullet
other firearms Y36.43-
patient is CIVILIAN Y36.431-
patient is MILITARY PERSONNEL Y36.430-
pellets Y36.42-
patient is CIVILIAN Y36.421-
patient is MILITARY PERSONNEL Y36.420-
E
Explosion (of) Y36.20- - *see also* Bomb, Detonation and Fragments
after cessation of hostilities Y36.8-
mine Y36.81-
patient is CIVILIAN Y36.810-
patient is MILITARY PERSONNEL Y36.811-
bomb Y36.82-
Patient is CIVILIAN Y36.821-
Patient is MILITARY PERSONNEL Y36.820-
artillery shell (sea based) Y36.03-
patient is CIVILIAN Y36.031-
patient is MILITARY PERSONNEL Y36.030-
depth-charge Y36.01-
patient is CIVILIAN Y36.011-
patient is MILITARY PERSONNEL Y36.010-
grenade Y36.29-
patient is CIVILIAN Y36.291-
patient is MILITARY PERSONNEL Y36.290-
guided missile Y36.22-
patient is CIVILIAN Y36.221-
patient is MILITARY PERSONNEL Y36.220-
improvised explosive device [IED] (person-borne) (roadside) (vehicle-borne) Y36.23-
patient is CIVILIAN Y36.231-
patient is MILITARY PERSONNEL Y36.230-
land mine Y36.29-
patient is CIVILIAN Y36.291-
patient is MILITARY PERSONNEL Y36.290-
marine mine (at sea) (in harbor) Y36.02-
patient is CIVILIAN Y36.021-
patient is MILITARY PERSONNEL Y36.020-

E (continued)
Explosion (of) Y36.20- - *see also* Bomb, Detonation and Fragments (continued)
marine weapon Y36.00-
accidental detonation of onboard weapon Y36.05-
patient is CIVILIAN Y36.051-
patient is MILITARY PERSONNEL Y36.050-
other specified – *see also* specific weapon Y36.09-
patient is CIVILIAN Y36.091-
patient is MILITARY PERSONNEL Y36.090-
unspecified marine weapon Y36.00-
patient is CIVILIAN Y36.001-
patient is MILITARY PERSONNEL Y36.000-
munitions or munitions launch device (accidental) Y36.24-
patient is CIVILIAN Y36.241-
patient is MILITARY PERSONNEL Y36.240-
F
Fire Y36.30- *see also* Flamethrower
specified fire NEC Y36.39-
patient is CIVILIAN Y36.391-
patient is MILITARY PERSONNEL Y36.390-
unspecified fire NOS Y36.30-
patient is CIVILIAN Y36.301-
patient is MILITARY PERSONNEL Y36.300-
Firearms – *see* Discharge (firearms)
Flamethrower Y36.33-
patient is CIVILIAN Y36.331-
patient is MILITARY PERSONNEL Y36.330-
Fragments (from) (of)
improvised explosive device [IED] (person-borne) (roadside) (vehicle-borne) Y36.26-
patient is CIVILIAN Y36.261-
patient is MILITARY PERSONNEL Y36.260-
munitions Y36.25-
patient is CIVILIAN Y36.251-
patient is MILITARY PERSONNEL Y36.250-
specified NEC Y36.29-
patient is CIVILIAN Y36.291--
patient is MILITARY PERSONNEL Y36.290-
weapons Y36.27-
patient is CIVILIAN Y36.271-
patient is MILITARY PERSONNEL Y36.270-
Friendly fire Y36.92-

These codes are used for injuries involving a patient who is either in the military or a civilian in a military setting. Injury occurred during a war, civil insurrection or peacekeeping mission. See also Military operations.

Military, War Operations, Gas to Other specified means

MILITARY, War Operations

G				N (continued)			
Gas – *see* Chemical weapons				**Nuclear weapon (effects of)** Y36.50- (continued)			
Gasoline bomb – *see* Bomb					indirect blast Y36.52-		
Grenade – *see* Explosion						patient is CIVILIAN Y36.521-	
Guided missile – *see* Explosion						patient is MILITARY PERSONNEL Y36.520-	
H					nuclear radiation Y36.54-		
Hand to hand (unarmed) combat Y36.44-						patient is CIVILIAN Y36.541-	
	patient is CIVILIAN Y36.441-					patient is MILITARY PERSONNEL Y36.540-	
	patient is MILITARY PERSONNEL Y36.440-				secondary effects Y36.54-		
Hot substances Y36.30-						patient is CIVILIAN Y36.541-	
	specified substance NEC Y36.39-					patient is MILITARY PERSONNEL Y36.540-	
		patient is CIVILIAN Y36.391-			specified effects NEC Y36.59-		
		patient is MILITARY PERSONNEL Y36.390-				patient is CIVILIAN Y36.591-	
	unspecified substance NOS Y36.30-					patient is MILITARY PERSONNEL Y36.590-	
		patient is CIVILIAN Y36.301-			thermal radiation Y36.53-		
		patient is MILITARY PERSONNEL Y36.300-				patient is CIVILIAN Y36.531-	
I						patient is MILITARY PERSONNEL Y36.530-	
Incendiary bullet – *see* Bullet					unspecified effects Y36.50-		
L						patient is CIVILIAN Y36.501-	
Land mine – *see* Explosion, bomb						patient is MILITARY PERSONNEL Y36.500-	
M				O			
Marine mine – *see* Explosion, marine weapon				**Object** – *see* Blunt or Piercing object			
Mine NOS – *see* Explosion				**Other specified means** Y36.90-			
Mortar bomb – *see* Bomb, unspecified					after cessation of hostilities		
Munitions – *see* Explosion						mine Y36.81-	
N							patient is CIVILIAN Y36.811-
Nuclear weapon (effects of) Y36.50-							patient is MILITARY PERSONNEL Y36.810-
	acute radiation exposure – *see* Nuclear radiation					bomb Y36.82-	
	direct blast Y36.51-						patient is CIVILIAN Y36.821-
		patient is CIVILIAN Y36.511-					patient is MILITARY PERSONNEL Y36.820-
		patient is MILITARY PERSONNEL Y36.510-				other Y36.88-	
	direct heat – *see* Nuclear weapon, thermal radiation						patient is CIVILIAN Y36.881-
	fallout exposure – *see* Nuclear weapon, nuclear radiation						patient is MILITARY PERSONNEL Y36.880-
	fireball (ionizing radiation) (immediate exposure) Y36.53-					unspecified Y36.89-	
		patient is CIVILIAN Y36.531-					patient is CIVILIAN Y36.891-
		patient is MILITARY PERSONNEL Y36.530-					patient is MILITARY PERSONNEL Y36.890-

These codes are used for injuries involving a patient who is either in the military or a civilian. Injury occurred during a war, civil insurrection or peacekeeping mission. See also Military operations.

Military, War Operations, Petrol bomb to Weapons

MILITARY, War Operations

P
Petrol bomb – see Fire
Phosgene – see Chemical weapons
Piercing (cutting) object Y36.45-
patient is CIVILIAN Y36.451-
patient is MILITARY PERSONNEL Y36.450-
R
Restriction of air (airway) (choking)
intentional (on purpose) Y36.46-
patient is CIVILIAN Y36.461-
patient is MILITARY PERSONNEL Y36.460-
unintentional (accidental) Y36.47-
patient is CIVILIAN Y36.471-
patient is MILITARY PERSONNEL Y36.470-

S
Sarin – see Chemical weapons
Shot down (aircraft) – see Destruction, aircraft
Shrapnel NOS Y36.29- see also Fragments
Smallpox – see Biological weapons
Stabbing – see Piercing instrument
Suffocation —see Restriction of airways
T
Torpedo – see Explosion, marine weapon
U
Underwater blast NOS Y36.00-
patient is CIVILIAN Y36.001-
patient is MILITARY PERSONNEL Y36.000-
Unconventional warfare NEC Y36.7X- see also Chemical and Biological warfare
patient is CIVILIAN Y36.7X1-
patient is MILITARY PERSONNEL Y36.7X0-
Unspecified means Y36.9-
W
Warfare
conventional NEC – see Conventional warfare
unconventional NEC – see Unconventional warfare
Weapons
biological – see Biological weapons
chemical – see Chemical weapons
nuclear – see Nuclear weapons (effects of)
specified NEC Y36.90-
weapon of mass destruction [WMD] Y36.91-

List intent/cause codes before other External Cause codes. Use more than one code if needed to completely explain the circumstances. **Use these codes throughout treatment With applicable 7th character.**

END OF INJURY, DURING WAR OPERATIONS

CATEGORY – INTENT/CAUSE MEDICAL TREATMENT/COMPLICATIONS
Adverse Incidents Associated with Devices

Type of Device	Type of Device
Anesthesiology device Y70.8	**Hospital (general) device** Y74.8 – *see also* surgical device
accessory Y70.2	accessory Y74.2
diagnostic Y70.0	diagnostic Y74.0
miscellaneous (other devices) Y70.8	miscellaneous (other devices) Y74.8
monitoring Y70.0	monitoring Y74.0
other implants Y70.2	other implants Y74.2
prosthetic Y70.2	prosthetic Y74.2
rehabilitative Y70.1	rehabilitative Y74.1
surgical instruments and materials (sutures) Y70.3	surgical instruments and materials Y74.3
therapeutic (nonsurgical) device Y70.1	therapeutic (nonsurgical) Y74.1
Cardiovascular device Y71.8	**Medical (nonsurgical) device** Y82.9 – *see also* type of device, therapeutic
accessory Y71.2	specified type NEC Y82.8
diagnostic Y71.0	**Neurological device** Y75.8
miscellaneous (other devices) Y71.8	accessory Y75.2
monitoring Y71.0	diagnostic Y75.0
other implants Y71.2	miscellaneous (other devices) Y75.8
prosthetic Y71.2	monitoring Y75.0
rehabilitative Y71.1	other implants Y75.2
surgical instruments and materials (sutures) Y71.3	prosthetic Y75.2
therapeutic (nonsurgical) device Y71.1	rehabilitative Y75.1
Ear – *see* Otorhinolaryngological device	surgical instruments and materials (sutures) Y75.3
Gastroenterology device Y73.8	therapeutic (nonsurgical) Y75.1
accessory Y73.2	**Nonsurgical device** – see medical device
diagnostic Y73.0	**Nose** – see Otorhinolaryngological device
miscellaneous (other device) Y73.8	**Obstetrical device** Y76.8
monitoring Y73.0	accessory Y76.2
other implants Y73.2	diagnostic Y76.0
prosthetic Y73.2	miscellaneous (other devices) Y76.8
rehabilitative Y73.1	monitoring Y76.0
surgical instruments and materials (sutures) Y73.3	other implants Y76.2
therapeutic (nonsurgical) Y73.1	prosthetic Y76.2
General device – see Adverse incidents due to medical device, hospital (general) or surgical (general)	rehabilitative Y76.1
Gynecological device Y76.8	surgical instruments and materials (sutures) Y76.3
accessory Y76.2	therapeutic (nonsurgical) Y76.1
diagnostic Y76.0	**Ophthalmic device** Y77.8
miscellaneous (other devices) Y76.8	accessory Y77.2
monitoring Y76.0	contact lens (rigid gas permeable) (soft) (hydrophilic) Y77.11
other implants Y76.2	diagnostic Y77.0
prosthetic Y76.2	miscellaneous (other devices) Y77.8
rehabilitative Y76.1	monitoring Y77.0
surgical instruments and materials (sutures) Y76.3	other implants Y77.2
therapeutic (nonsurgical) Y76.1	prosthetic Y77.2
	rehabilitative Y77.19
	surgical instruments and materials (sutures) Y77.3
	therapeutic (nonsurgical) Y77.19

Code also complication codes Y83-&84 or misadventure &62-Y69 if appropriate.

Medical, Adverse incidents, Orthopedic to Urology device

MEDICAL TREATMENT/COMPLICATIONS
Adverse incidents Associated with Device

Type of Device	Type of Device
Orthopedic device (internal fixation device) Y79.8 *see also* Physical medicine device	**Plastic surgical device** Y81.8
accessory Y79.2	accessory Y81.2
diagnostic Y79.0	diagnostic Y81.0
miscellaneous (other instruments) Y79.8	miscellaneous (other devices) Y81.8
monitoring Y79.0	monitoring Y81.0
other implants 79.2	other implants Y81.2
prosthetic Y79.2	prosthetic Y81.2
rehabilitative Y79.1	rehabilitative Y81.1
surgical instruments and materials (sutures) Y79.3	surgical instruments and materials (sutures) Y81.3
therapeutic (nonsurgical) Y79.1	therapeutic (nonsurgical) Y81.1
Otorhinolaryngological device Y72.8	**Radiological device** Y78.8
accessory Y72.2	accessory Y78.2
diagnostic Y72.0	diagnostic Y78.0
miscellaneous (other devices) Y72.8	miscellaneous (other devices) Y78.8
monitoring Y72.0	monitoring Y78.0
other implants Y72.2	other implants Y78.2
prosthetic Y72.2	prosthetic Y78.2
rehabilitative Y72.1	rehabilitative Y78.1
surgical instruments and materials (sutures) Y72.3	surgical instruments and materials (sutures) Y78.3
therapeutic (nonsurgical) Y72.1	therapeutic (nonsurgical) Y78.1
Personal use device Y74.8	**Surgical (general) device** (nonhospital) Y81.8 - *see also* hospital (general) device
accessory Y74.2	accessory Y80.2
diagnostic Y74.0	diagnostic Y81.0
miscellaneous (other devices) Y74.8	miscellaneous (other devices) Y81.8
monitoring Y74.0	monitoring Y81.0
other implants Y74.2	other implants Y81.2
prosthetic Y74.2	prosthetic Y81.2
rehabilitative Y74.1	rehabilitative Y81.1
surgical instruments and materials (sutures) Y74.3	surgical instruments and materials (sutures) Y81.3
therapeutic (nonsurgical) Y74.1	therapeutic Y81.1
Physical medicine device (cane, powered wheelchair) Y80.8 - *see also* orthopedic devices	**Throat device** – see Otorhinolaryngological device
	Urology device Y73.8
accessory Y80.2	accessory Y73.2
diagnostic Y80.0	diagnostic Y73.0
miscellaneous (other devices) Y80.8	miscellaneous (other devices) Y73.8
monitoring Y80.0	monitoring Y73.0
other implants Y80.2	other implants Y73.2
prosthetic Y80.2	prosthetic Y73.2
rehabilitative Y80.1	rehabilitative Y73.1
surgical instruments and materials (sutures) Y80.3	surgical instruments and materials (sutures) Y73.3
	therapeutic (nonsurgical) Y73.1

Use more than one complication code if appropriate.
Use these codes throughout treatment with applicable 7th character.

END ADVERSE INCIDENTS

CATEGORY – INTENT/CAUSE MEDICAL TREATMENT/COMPLICATIONS
Complication of Medical or Surgical Procedures

Medical Procedures (Nonsurgical) Y84
Aspiration (of)
fluid Y84.4-
tissue Y84.8
Biopsy Y84.8
Blood
sampling Y84.7
transfusion Y84.8
Breakdown of device – see Adverse incident, device
Bypass Y83.2
Catheterization
cardiac Y84.0
urinary Y84.6
Dialysis (kidney) Y84.1
Drug —see Table of Drugs and Chemicals
Duodenal sound (probe) (insertion of) Y84.5
Electroshock therapy Y84.3
Gastric sound (probe) (insertion of) Y84.5
Infusion procedure Y84.8
Injection procedure Y84.8
drug injected - see Table of Drugs and Chemicals
Insertion of gastric or duodenal sound (probe) Y84.5
Insulin-shock therapy Y84.3
Late effects – see Sequelae
Paracentesis (abdominal) (thoracic) Y84.4
Medical device – see Adverse incident, device
Radiological procedure Y84.2
Radiotherapy Y84.2
Sampling
blood Y84.7
fluid NEC Y84.4
tissue Y84.8
Shock therapy V84.3
Sound (probe) (insertion of) Y84.5
duodenal Y84.5
gastric Y84.5
Sequelae (late effects) – use code for original injury with 7th character S
Transfusion Y84.8
complication due to substance being transfused - see Table of Drugs and Chemicals
complication due to transfusion procedure Y84.8
Other medical procedure Y84.8
Unspecified medical procedure Y84.9
Vaccination Y84.8
complication due to drug administered - see Table of Drugs and Chemicals
complication due to vaccination procedure V84.8

Surgical Operation/Procedure Y83
Amputation Y83.5
Anastomosis Y83.2
Bypass Y83.2
Colostomy Y83.3
Cystostomy Y83.3
Duodenostomy Y83.3
Electrodes in brain Y83.1
External stoma, creation of Y83.3
Formation of external stoma Y83.3
Gastrostomy Y83.3
Graft Y83.2
Heart valve prosthesis Y83.1
Hemorrhage —see Index to Diseases and Injuries, complication(s)
Hypothermia (medically-induced) (complication of) Y84.8
Implant, implantation – see Abnormal reaction
Incident, adverse, due to medical devices – see Adverse reaction
Late effects – see Sequelae
Other internal device Y83.1
Other opening to outside body (stoma) Y83.3
Other surgical procedure Y83.8
Pacemaker Y83.1
Perforation - see Index to Disease and Injuries, complications
Procedure, reaction to – see Abnormal reaction
Reconstructive surgery NEC (with) Y83.4
anastomosis, bypass or graft Y83.2
formation of external stoma Y83.3
specified NEC Y83.8
Removal of organ (partial) (total) Y83.6
Sequelae (late effects) – use code for original injury with 7th character S
Transplant of organ (whole) Y83.0
partial Y83.4
Unspecified surgical procedure Y83.9

Code also breakdown or malfunction of device (Y70-Y82) if appropriate

Use these codes throughout treatment with appropriate 7th character.

END OF COMPLICATIONS CODES

CATEGORY – INTENT/CAUSE MEDICAL TREATMENT/COMPLICATIONS
Misadventures

A
Anesthesia
failure to introduce endotracheal tube Y65.4
wrong placement of endotracheal tube Y65.3
Aspiration of fluid or tissue (by puncture or catheterization except heart)
failure of sterile precautions Y62.6
B
Biologicals —*see also* Table of Drugs and Chemicals
needle (aspirating) failure of sterile precautions Y62.6
Biopsy (except needle aspiration) failure of sterile precautions Y62.8
needle (aspirating) failure of sterile precautions Y62.6
Blood
contaminated (administered by) (administered for) Y64.9
immunization Y64.1
infusion Y64.0
injection Y64.1
other specified means of administration Y64.8
transfusion Y64.0
unspecified means of administration Y64.9
vaccination Y64.1
mismatched (in transfusion) V65.0
C
Catheterization (failure of sterile precautions during)
heart catheterization Y62.5
other catheterization Y62.6
removal of catheter Y62.8
D
Dialysis (kidney) failure of sterile precautions Y62.2
Drugs —*see also* Table of Drugs and Chemicals
contaminated (administered by) Y64.9
immunization Y64.1
infusion Y64.0
injection Y64.1
other specified means of administration Y64.8
transfusion Y64.0
unspecified means of administration Y64.9
vaccination Y64.1
incorrect dosage (during) Y63.9
excessive (transfusion or infusion) Y63.0-
Incorrect dilution (infusion) Y63.1-
Insulin-shock therapy Y63.4-
specified surgical or medical care Y63.8
unspecified surgical or medical care Y63.9
not administered (drug necessary) Y63.6
overdose —*see* Table of Drugs and Chemicals
underdose – Y63.3-

E
Electroshock therapy (incorrect dosage) Y63.4
Endoscopic examination, failure of sterile precautions Y62.4
Endotracheal tube (in anesthesia)
failure to introduce endotracheal tube Y65.4
failure to remove endotracheal tube Y65.4
wrong placement of endotracheal tube Y65.3
F
Failure – *see also* specific procedure
sterile precautions (during procedure) NEC Y62.8
sterile precautions (during procedure) NOS Y62.9
suture or ligature during surgical procedure Y65.2
to introduce tube or instrument Y65.4
endotracheal tube during anesthesia Y65.3
failure to remove tube or instrument Y65.4
Fluids (other than blood or drugs)
contaminated (administered by) Y64.9
immunization Y64.1
infusion Y64.0
injection Y64.1
other specified means of administration Y64.8
transfusion Y64.0
unspecified means of administration Y64.9
vaccination Y64.1
excessive amount of fluid given Y63.0
failure of sterile precautions Y62.1
immunization, failure of sterile precautions Y62.3
incorrect dilution of fluid given Y63.1
injection Y62.3
wrong fluid given Y65.1
H
Heart catheterization, failure of sterile precautions Y62.5
I
Immunization – contaminated drug Y64.1
Inappropriate – *see* Wrong
Infusion
contaminated blood or drug given Y64.0
excessive amount of blood or fluid given Y63.0
failure of sterile precautions Y62.1
incorrect dilution of fluid Y63.1
overdose —*see* Table of Drugs and Chemicals
wrong fluid given Y65.1
Injection
contaminated blood or drug given Y64.1
failure of sterile precautions Y62.3
insulin-shock therapy (incorrect dosage) Y63.4

Code also adverse incident due to device Y70-Y82 if appropriate.

INTENT/CAUSE MEDICAL TREATMENT/COMPLICATIONS
Misadventures

K	
Kidney dialysis – failure of sterile precautions Y62.2	

L	
Ligation failure (during surgical procedure) Y65.2	
lumbar puncture, failure of sterile precautions Y62.6	

M	
Mismatched blood (in transfusion) V65.0	

N	
Nonadministration	
	drug (necessary) not given Y63.6
	surgical or medical care not provided or ended prematurely (too early) Y66
Nosocomial condition Y95	

O	
Other mechanical, of instrument or apparatus (any) (during any procedure) Y65.8	
Overdose —see Drugs, Table of Drugs and Chemicals	
	during specified procedure NEC Y63.8
Other specified misadventure Y65.8	

P	
Packing	
	failure of sterile precautions Y62.8
	too hot or too cold Y63.5
Paracentesis (abdominal) (thoracic), failure of sterile precautions Y62.6	
Perforation —see Index to Diseases and Injuries, Complications	
Perfusion, failure of sterile precautions Y62.2	
Puncture - see Index to Diseases and Injuries	
Procedure (wrong procedure performed) – see Wrong	

R	
Radiotherapy Y63.2	
	inadvertent (accidental) exposure of patient (receiving test or therapy) Y63.3
	overdose (in medical or surgical procedure) V63.2

S	
Scalding from externally applied substance Y63.5	
Sterile precautions (during procedure) (failure of) - see also specific procedure	
	specified procedure NEC Y62.8
	surgical operation Y62.0
	unspecified procedure Y62.9
Surgical instrument (failure to introduce or remove) Y65.4	
Suture failure (during surgical procedure) Y65.2	

T	
Temperature – inappropriate (too hot or too cold) in local application and packing Y63.5	
Tube – see also Endotracheal tube or Endoscopic exam	
	failure to introduce or remove tube Y65.4
Transfusion	
	contaminated blood or drug given Y64.0
	excessive amount of blood or other fluid given Y63.0
	failure sterile precautions Y62.1
	mismatched blood Y65.0

U	
Underdosing of necessary drugs, medicaments or biological substances Y63.6	
Unspecified misadventure Y69	

V	
Vaccination	
	contaminated drug given Y64.1-
	vaccine —see Table of Drugs and Chemicals
	procedure, failure of sterile precautions Y62.3

W	
Wrong	
	blood (mismatched) in infusion Y65.0
	device (correct procedure but wrong device) Y65.51
	fluid used in infusion Y65.1
	right patient, wrong procedure Y65.51
	wrong patient Y65.52
	procedure performed Y65.51
	side or part of body (correct procedure, wrong side or body part) Y65.53

List intent/cause codes before other External Cause codes. Use more than one code if needed to completely explain circumstances.

Use these codes throughout treatment with applicable 7th character.

END OF MEDICAL TREATMENT/COMPLICATIONS, MISADVENTURES

SEQUELA

Sequela (of) (after effect) (condition that is result of previous (treated) disease or (healed) injury) Listed by original injury which resulted in sequela	
Accident NEC —*see* W00-X58 with 7th character S	**Legal intervention** - *see* Y35 with 7th character S
Air and space craft – *see* V95-V99 with 7th character S	**Military operations** – *see* Y37 with 7th character S
Assault (homicidal) (any means) —*see* X92-Y09 with 7th character S if available	**Misadventures** – *see* Y62-Y69 with 7th character S if available
	Motor vehicle accident —*see* V00-V99 with 7th character S
Homicide, attempt (any means) —*see* X92-Y09 with 7th character S	**Suicide, attempt** (any means) —*see* X71-X83 with 7th character S
	Watercraft – *see* V90-V94 with 7th character S
Injury undetermined - see Y21-U33 with 7th character S	
Intentional self-harm —*see* X71-X83 with 7th character S	

SUPPLEMENTAL FACTORS

Supplemental factors – Blood alcohol levels Y90	
Blood alcohol level Y90.9	
	less than 20 mg/100 ml Y90.0
	presence in blood, level not specified Y90.9
	20-39 mg/100 ml Y90.1
	40-59 mg/100 ml Y90.2
	60-79 mg/100 ml Y90.3
	80-99 mg/100 ml Y90.4
	100-119 mg/100 ml Y90.5
	120-199 mg/100 ml Y90.6
	200-239 mg/100 ml Y90.7
	240 mg/100 ml or more Y90.8

Other Books by Terry Tropin

ICD-10-CM Coding Guidelines Made Easy

ICD-10-PCS Coding Guidelines Made Easy

Evaluation and Management Coding Made Easy

Look for annual updates of these books!

Visit me on Facebook – Tropin's Medical Coding, https://www.facebook.com/codingteacher

Made in the USA
Middletown, DE
08 March 2021